YOUR PATH TO
HEALTHIER DENTISTRY

YOUR PATH TO HEALTHIER DENTISTRY

*a holistic approach to keeping
your teeth for a lifetime*

Dr. Alex Shvartsman

ISBN: 978-1-4817-4118-7 (sc)
ISBN: 978-1-4817-4119-4 (e)

Library of Congress Control Number: 2013906745

For my son, Logan

*May you find a career as fulfilling
and rewarding as I have.*

CONTENTS

*In the future revisions of this book this chapter will see the most change. I look forward to moving the following sections to the previous chapter and fill the upcoming pages with new exciting advanced we can all look forward to.

INTRODUCTION

Today dentistry is changing at a rapid pace. It is a truly exciting time to be a dentist. However, it is an amazing time to be the patient. New advances in all disciplines of dentistry have made it possible to provide comfortable, esthetic, long lasting and healthy dental care.

It is also a scary time to be the patient. Globally and in the USA tooth decay and gum disease are on the rise. The impact of oral disease on the total heath of the body can no longer be denied or ignored.

Unfortunately the responsibility for your health falls on no one but you. Neither the government, insurance companies nor dental organizations have your best interests in mind. Do not fear, for in the following pages you will gain the knowledge of how to keep your teeth for a lifetime and become your own dental health care advocate. This book may make you laugh, shock you, anger you but most importantly it will empower you with knowledge to help you make better decisions about healthier dental care for you and your family.

DIAGNOSIS

In dentistry as in medicine, there is only one right diagnosis and many treatment options. With today's rapidly evolving technology, new dental diagnostic methods are available to improve our identification of oral disease. This chapter will explore this in further detail so you, the consumer can learn what to expect and ask for.

TOOTH DECAY DIAGNOSIS

Laser Cavity Detection

Traditionally dentists use a sharp-pointy pick to check for cavities. You may have had this instrument stuck in your tooth in the past. Not only can this be painful, but also a sharp-pointy instrument coming at your face is not a comforting experience if you are already nervous at the dentist. In addition, the sharp metal pick can damage weakened enamel and potentiate cavity formation. The fact is that cavity detection with this technique is at best only about 60% accurate; many small cavities go unseen and can become large cavities if left untreated. This can lead to unnecessary root canal treatment, crowns or extractions.

There are several tooth decay detection devices now available, the most widely used is the Diagnodent: the laser cavity detection system. This decay laser is over 90% effective in painlessly finding even the smallest cavities early, when they can be treated conservatively with a small filling.

Digital 2-D x-rays

There are many advantages of digital dental x-rays over conventional film x-rays. Digital x-rays use an electronic sensor to capture the image. Studies estimate that radiation exposure can be reduced by about 90% with digital dental x-rays. The best systems can reduce radiation by about 98%.

The image can be refined to improve and aid in dental diagnosis. The zoom-in feature allows dentists to see more detail. Contrast changing ability can help detect the smallest cavity as well as hidden tartar under the gums. Many current software systems have decay finding features to help point out small cavities. The image appears in a few seconds and can be displayed on a TV screen so patients can see their x-rays better. An additional benefit of this technology is that there is no environmental waste from chemicals, plastic and lead as there is with conventional dental film x-rays. A draw back to all 2-D x-rays is that they area two dimensional representation of a three dimensional object and are subject to interpretation. Decay is always bigger in real life than how it appears on 2-D x-rays.

Digital 3-D x-rays

Cone Beam Computed Tomography (CBCT) is a recent addition to dentistry's armamentarium. It is a powerful diagnostic tool, which allows dentists to finally look inside teeth and accurately evaluate the depth of cavities. Although currently not as sharp as 2-D dental x-rays this innovative diagnostic technology will improve with time and will someday replace 2-D x-rays.

Transillumination

Traditionally, decay between teeth (interproximal decay) is diagnosed by the use of dental x-rays. However, a new device to identify tooth decay in between the front teeth has become available. It uses a light instead of x-rays, allowing modern dentists to minimize their patients' radiation exposure. The transilluminator uses a strong beam of focused light to illuminate the front teeth. Since the front teeth are flat, they allow light to go directly though them. Transillumination used by an experienced dentist can pick up even small cavities between the front teeth.

GUM DISEASE DIAGNOSIS

Very little has changed in the way dentists evaluate patients for the presence of gum disease. Although the standard of care is a full gum disease evaluation once a year, according to the American Academy of Periodontics few dentists actually do this routinely. The periodontal exam consists of x-ray evaluation to see the level of supporting bone around the teeth and measuring the space between the gum and the tooth with a round-ended ruler called "perio probing". As well as evaluating the color, shape, quality and recession of gums and noting areas of heavy bleeding. In addition, some dentists use a phase contrast microscope to assay the type and amount of bacteria under the gums. This helps dentists to custom tailor treatment based on the microorganisms infecting the gums. This leads to more effective gum disease treatment.

ORAL CANCER DIAGNOSIS

Every hour of every day, one American dies of oral cancer. The mortality rate associated with oral cancer has not improved significantly in the last 40 years. More than 30,000 Americans will receive an oral cancer diagnosis this year. In five years, only 57% will still be alive. 27% of oral cancer victims do not use tobacco or alcohol and have no other lifestyle risk factors.

Oral cancer is one of the most curable diseases when it's caught early. Several new non-invasive oral inspection tests have been developed to screen for oral cancer. Lights of different wavelengths are used with special filtering glasses to identify and further evaluate suspicious areas of the mouth. Similar technology has proven successful in identifying soft tissue abnormalities in other areas of the body. One device in particular combines all the available lights and provides a comprehensive oral screening procedure for patients at increased risk for oral cancer. The Trimera Identifi 3000 exam is painless, fast, and helps dentists to see abnormal tissue that is not visible to the naked eye during a routine exam.

A brush biopsy-screening test is another useful tool. Suspicious areas of the mouth can be lightly brushed with a specially designed stiff bristle brush to collect cells. The specimen is sent to a lab to look for pre-cancerous or cancerous cells.

Minimally invasive oral cancer technologies can help identify early mouth cancers without the need for invasive biopsies, which require cutting, stitching, and discomfort for several days to weeks.

BAD BREATH DIAGNOSIS

While there are many causes of bad breath, one major contributor are *Volatile Sulfur Compounds*

(VSC's). Two sulfur-containing amino acids, cisteine and methionine, found in protein are the main source of VSC's. Patients with high levels of VSC's tend to get very bad breath. A machine called the Halorimeter can be used to detect the presence of these compounds. Recently, a product has been developed that looks like a q-tip and can be used to detect the presence of VSC's in a few seconds by swabbing the gums.

New technologies are emerging that will make dental diagnosis better and help improve the care of patients.

PREVENTION

Prevention of disease is the key to continued good health. This is the most important chapter in this book. So pay attention!

The old saying "an ounce is prevention is worth a pound of cure" rings true to this day. Except in cases of trauma, every crown, root canal and tooth extracted because of tooth decay all began as a tiny cavity. Had that cavity been diagnosed early, it could have been treated in a conservative, minimally invasive and least expensive manner. Since small cavities and gum disease are typically painless, people are initially unaware of any problems in their mouth.

People who avoid the dentist for professional cleanings and exams are really short changing themselves. Years can go by without any symptoms. Finally when a tooth breaks because the cavity has undermined and weakened the tooth or pain sets in because the decay has reached the nerve, the amount of tooth destruction can be massive. The cost associated with restoring the tooth is now 10 to 20 times more than it would have been had the cavity been diagnosed when it was tiny. Worse, however is the actual tooth destruction that has occurred. As advanced as dentistry is today, nothing is as good or as strong as your own natural teeth. The key to keeping your teeth for a lifetime is to keep as much of your own natural, healthy teeth for a lifetime. Nothing man-made is better than nature.

The college syndrome

When young people leave the protective nest and go away to school, typically their dental health suffers. Late nights of studying are usually accompanied by coffee, soda and energy drinks (more on that later). Junk food made with processed and refined carbohydrates becomes the norm and not the exception. Gone are the parents who nag them to brush their teeth before going to bed. Combined with a lack of flossing, results in an increased tooth decay rate. It is not uncommon to see kids coming back from college with a mouth riddled with cavities.

To make matters worse, going to the dentist for a professional exam and a cleaning becomes and after thought when they return from college during vacation. Typically, a college student comes in at the very end of their break and not at the very beginning. When problems are diagnosed, there is usually no time to treat them because the student is leaving for college within a few days or the next day! Months can go by until they return for treatment. By then the cavities are much bigger, more costly to treat and have destroyed more of the natural healthy tooth. If you do nothing else, please make sure to see the dentist at the beginning of the college break and not the end.

The no insurance syndrome

Many people avoid the dentist because of a lack of dental insurance. This is common with young adults when they come off their parents insurance and do not have a job that provides dental coverage. By avoiding regular professional cleanings and exams, small cavities and early gum disease silently progress and do their damage. By the time the person finally sees a dentist the amount of tooth destruction and the cost of treating it may be daunting. The money saved by not going to the dentist for exams and cleanings pales in comparison to the cost of treatment. It is not only cost effective to invest in regular check-ups, but it is less tooth destructive as well.

TOOTH DECAY PREVENTION

Diet

You may not realize this, but tooth decay was virtually non-existent over 10,000 years ago. Tooth decay is a human made disease. Our pets and us are the only animals on this planet that develop tooth decay. In fact, tooth decay is a relatively modern disease, first seen in the archeological record with the advent of grain consumption, which led to farming. Tooth decay as well as many other diseases are what used to be called "diseases of civilization", until it became politically incorrect. However, it is a very fitting name and it includes cardio-vascular disease, strokes, heart attacks, many cancers, obesity, high blood pressure, diabetes, food allergies, and autoimmune diseases such as Lupus, Alzheimer's, multiple sclerosis, Type I diabetes, vetiligo, psoriasis, etc.

After about 250,000 living as hunter-gatherers, approximately 10,000 years ago humans began transitioning to a life of farming. Agriculture has turned out to be a double edge sword. It allowed humans to develop civilization and technology at the expense of our health. Today at the highest point of human civilization and technological achievement we are sicker than we have ever been before and it is going to get worse! We went form a diet that we evolved to eat for 2 million years, a diet that gave us our large and impressive brain, to a diet that, in the short 10,000 years of agriculture and processed foods, is full of foods that are foreign to our body and metabolism.

We evolved eating a diet of meat, fish, poultry (and the natural fat that came along with these animals) and seasonal veggies and fruit. Skeletons of our ancestors showed perfectly straight teeth with zero cavities. These skeletons also showed people with strong robust bones with muscle insertions similar to today's top athletes. Of the little over 200 remaining pockets of hunter-gatherers left today none of these people show any signs of tooth decay or any other disease of civilization.

Our agricultural diet is full of foods that we are not designed to eat. These foods include grains, legumes, dairy, plant oils, sugar and exorbitant levels of fructose found in processed food and unnaturally sweet fruit that are available to us year round and not just in summer and autumn as is natural. The abnormally enormous levels of carbohydrates as well as anti-nutrients and toxins found in these "evolutionarily foreign" foods are making us sicker and sicker.

Seeds such as grains and legumes are the "babies" of plants. Since plants have no claws, teeth or legs the only defense against their seeds being eaten is biologic chemical warfare: toxins and anti-nutrients. Enough of these chemicals survive heating and digestion to wreak havoc on our health. While nuts also have some levels of toxins, it is far less due their primary defense: a hard wooden shell.

Dairy is also an unnatural food. We are the only mammals on this planet that drink the milk of other mammals into adult hood. No wonder most of the world's human population is lactose intolerant. Milk makes babies grow, and cow babies need to grow FAST! Not only is milk loaded with proteins that are toxic and allergic to humans, it is full of natural (and often added) growth hormones.

Plant oils are loaded with omega 6 fatty acids that are pro-inflammatory and create an unnaturally high omega 6:omega 3 ratio in our diet. Fruits have been bred to be large, sweet, lower in fiber and are now available all year round. Together with High Fructose Corn Syrup found in everything from ketchup to salad dressing we are overloading our liver with fructose and destroying our health and teeth.

So if you want to stop cavities and cure yourself from "diseases of civilization", begin eating and moving like our Paleolithic ancestors did. For further reading on this subject you may want to read: The Paleolithic Solution by Robb Wolf, Primal Blueprint by Mark Sisson, The Paleo Diet (2010 edition) and Palo Answer by Lauren Cordain.

Modern Cavity Prevention

If you are unwilling or unable to eat like our ancestors, there are modern ways to help prevent and reverse tooth decay, an oral disease that has plagued people for the past 10,000 years. It is said knowledge is power, so first let's understand how cavities form and then how to prevent them based on the latest research and prevention methods.

In order to get tooth decay three things are needed: Teeth, Bacteria, and Sugar. Teeth are what we want to keep and make acid and decay resistant. Plaque is the white soft deposit that forms daily on our teeth. Plaque is full of billions of bacteria that cause dental disease. Some bacteria infect our teeth and cause cavities, some infect our gums and jaw bone and cause gum disease. Sugar is what bacteria eat and produce the acid that they use to dissolve our teeth, causing cavities. Of note is that all carbohydrates break down to sugar in your mouth and as far as decay causing bacteria is concerned are the same as sugar.

SUGAR: As we continue to eat progressively refined starchy and processed food, tooth decay has become a global epidemic. As refined carbohydrates became more available and as our food industry began replacing fat with carbohydrates during the "fat phobia craze" in the past decades, tooth decay has become more prevalent. You can either return to a hunter-gatherer way of eating (meats, vegetables, and seasonal fruit and nuts), or focus on chemical means of prevention.

BACTERIA: Daily removal of dental plaque is a must. Bacterial plaque forms around your teeth within 24 hours after brushing and flossing. Using an electric toothbrush like the Oral B Triumph with its small head that can reach the back teeth is a great option for those that have a high gag reflex.

Teeth have 5 cleanable surfaces. Brushing cleans only 3 surfaces (the top, the tongue side and the cheek side). Not flossing is like not cleaning 2/5th of your teeth. Imagine taking a shower and only washing the top of your head, the front and the back of your body and never washing the sides. You would get stinky pretty quickly! Now you know how your teeth feel. Use shred-free floss, like Glide or Satin floss, which makes the flossing process much easier.

Another way to reduce the bacterial load in your mouth is by using xylitol. This natural sugar alcohol is toxic to decay causing bacteria and has been proven to reduce decay. Xylitol comes in gum and mints as well as granular powder that can be added to foods and drinks. It has a low glycemic index and is safe for diabetics. Look for 100% xylitol products. In addition, oil pulling, an Aurvedic technique, thousands of years old, has also been shown to reduce tooth decay susceptability.

TEETH: Although fluoride is very controversial (more on that later), this natural mineral needs be mentioned as part of a decay reduction discussion.

When applied directly to teeth, fluoride helps to reverse enamel cavities and creates a decay resistant outer layer on our teeth. Prescription strength pastes are available as well as over the counter rinses. If you decide to use a fluoride rinse or toothpaste make sure not to eat, drink or rinse for 30 minutes following the use of these products. The best time to use fluoride rinses and toothpaste is right before bed.

If you are against using topical fluoride, fortunately there are two products that can help reverse small cavities. These products are strong remineralizing agents that contain amorphous calcium and phosphate (ACP) and create a powerful remineralization environment in your mouth. Recaldent is found in MI Paste and Novamin is found in Renew Paste. Both products are available thought your dentist and have been proven to reduce sensitivity and reverse early cavities. MI Paste comes in both fluoridated and a fluoride free version, while Renew Paste contains prescription strength fluoride as well as Novamin.

XYLITOL: Natures Cavity Fighter

Xylitol, a dietary substance long used in the management of diabetes and weight control, is proving to be a healthcare powerhouse. Repeated studies indicate this sugar substitute has strong cavity-fighting properties when used several times a day. Studies have also shown xylitol to reduce sinus and ear infections. There is no aftertaste and xylitol has only half the calories of table sugar. Xylitol also has an 88% slower absorption rate of sugar, helping to keep blood sugar levels stable making it a great choice for diabetics.

Xylitol is a sugar alcohol found in plants such as berries, corn and plums. It also is produced in humans during normal metabolism. Dental effects include inhibiting decay-causing bacteria from multiplying in the mouth. This therapeutic sweetener significantly reduces the decay causing bacteria Streptococcus mutans in the mouth. It lowers oral acid levels, adjusts pH and reduces tooth plaque, resulting in less tooth decay and gum disease. Frequent use of xylitol, whether in the form of gum, mints, toothpaste or oral wash appears to break the tooth decay cycle.

A yearlong study in Finland showed an 85% reduction in cavity rates for subjects who chewed gum containing 6-10 grams of xylitol each day. Similar tooth decay reduction was found in subjects who followed strict diet guidelines and used xylitol as a sugar substitute. Other studies found that dental plaque accumulation was reduced by about 50% in less than a week of xylitol use. Similar results were found in more recent studies in Russia, the United States, New Zealand, Thailand and Canada. A

Danish researcher has even correlated xylitol use by mothers with decreased tooth decay in babies.

Xylitol is safe for use in children as demonstrated by a 40-month, multi-national chewing gum study published in the Journal of Dental Research. The investigation showed decreased tooth decay for children chewing xylitol gum in comparison to those who chewed none or had gum sweetened with other substances. In a follow-up study five years later by the University of Washington, xylitol subjects showed a 70% reduction in tooth decay: evidence of long-term benefits.

The sweetener has been linked to tooth self-repair through increased calcium uptake from saliva, reduction in bacterial levels, improved saliva levels in dry mouth patients and reduced ear infection cases in children.

Additional benefits of xylitol include an increase in white blood cells, which are part of a body's natural defense against bacterial infections. Studies indicate that xylitol in the diet promotes the intestinal absorption of calcium and has the potential to reduce or reverse bone loss in humans. Its use is being considered as a preventive measure to deal with osteoporosis, which affects more than 10 million people in the United States.

Two of best gum and mints that have this active ingredient are Zellies and Epic. Both are 100% xylitol products. Please visit www.zellies.com for more information on xylitol.

Fluoride: Friend and Foe.
The Misunderstood Mineral.

The mention of the word "fluoride" sends shivers down the spines of most holistic people. The Internet is teaming with websites condemning fluoride. Many books have been written about its negative health effects.

There is no doubt that systemic fluoride is bad for our health and water fluoridation has been a disastrous government health experiment. Ingesting fluoride is dangerous for adults and may be more harmful for children. In November of 2006, the American Dental Association (ADA) advised that parents should avoid giving babies' fluoridated water due to increased risk of brain damage and other health effects. Ingestion of excessive fluoride during tooth development can lead to unaesthetic brown mottling and pitting of permanent teeth, a condition called fluorosis. In addition, fluorosis has been associated with lower IQ scores in children in a recent study. Adults ingesting fluoride get zero benefit for their teeth, but the health consequences can be devastating. Systemic fluoride has been implicated in neurological damage, reduced thyroid function, weakened bones, increased bone cancer risk, increased risk for arthritis, increased infertility in men and early onset puberty in women. Fluoride may be hidden in any man-made beverages such as soda, iced tea, beer, wine, sports drinks or energy drinks. Moreover, discontinuing water fluoridation has not shown to increase tooth decay risk.

The fact remains that when fluoride is applied directly to teeth there is a significant benefit against tooth decay. Globally, tooth decay rates are on the rise. Our consumption of ever increasing processed carbohydrates and sugar as well as bacteria mutating to more aggressive forms are the main reasons for this new epidemic. Fluoride can play a significant role in preventing and reversing tooth decay.

When applied directly to the teeth (topically), fluoride can help heal early cavities in the enamel. The healed enamel (fluorapatite) becomes highly acid resistant. Continued use of topically applied fluoride creates an acid resistant layer in both enamel and exposed tooth roots. Fluoride has also been effective in reducing tooth sensitivity.

The key question is "how much fluoride penetrates the skin of the mouth?" In other words, what is the systemic fluoride impact on a 1-minute fluoride rinse or brushing your teeth with prescription strength fluoride toothpaste for 2 minutes? It turns out that the there is no evidence that topically applied fluoride has any systemic effects.

It is important to understand that ingesting fluoride and tooth surface treatment with fluoride are two completely different and separate things. Lumping both together is irresponsible and shows a lack of knowledge. Perhaps it is time to rethink our demonization of fluoride as a whole and shun its systemic use, while embracing its topical benefits.

Drinks That Ruin Your Teeth
Although it is well known that sugar causes tooth decay, acid is an often-overlooked problem. Acidic drinks with sugar spells double trouble for your teeth. However even sugar-free drinks can cause took damage if they contain acid.

Approximately 40% of U.S. teenagers are consuming sports and energy drinks on a daily basis. It is important that parents and young adults as well as fitness enthusiasts understand the disadvantages these drinks can pose to oral health. Scientific studies are now revealing the full extent of damage a person can inadvertently cause to their tooth enamel by consuming highly acidic beverages.

People who pursue a healthy, active lifestyle ironically may avoid colas or sugary drinks in favor of what they believe to be a 'healthier' alternative and so they tend to rely on sports or energy drinks to rehydrate after exercising. The results of a recent study point to the fact that regular long-term use of such highly acidic beverages can lead to irreversible damage to tooth enamel.

From this and other similar studies it can now be concluded that the enamel damage associated with all acidic beverages ranging from greatest (1) to least (6) damage to dental enamel are as follows:

1. Lemonade
2. Energy drinks
3. Sports drinks
4. Fitness water
5. Sugar free soda
6. Unsweetened iced tea mix

Most cola-based drinks contain more than one type of acid, generally phosphoric and citric acids, both of which contribute to enamel damage. Sports beverages contain a range of other additives and organic acids that further worsen dental erosion. Organic acids also demineralize tooth enamel as they break down calcium, which is needed to strengthen teeth and prevent gum disease.

The best way to avoid damaging your dental enamel is to not drink sports drinks and similar beverages on a routine basis. The best choice to rehydrate is always plain water. If your goal is to replenish electrolytes after profuse sweating then unsweetened and unflavored plain coconut water can help to preserve tooth enamel and ultimately protect teeth from decay. If you must drink acidic beverages it is advisable to chew sugar-free gum or rinse the mouth with water following consumption of the drinks as a way to increase saliva flow, which naturally helps to normalize acidity levels in the mouth. In addition, in order to avoid spreading acid onto the tooth surfaces thereby increasing the erosive action, it is a good idea to wait at least an hour before brushing after consuming sports and energy drinks.

GUM DISEASE PREVENTION

Gum disease or periodontal disease is a silent epidemic in the US. Studies estimate that nearly 85% of the population has some stage of gum disease. In addition, approximately 50% of the people fall into the moderate to severe classification. In fact, gum disease is the # 1 reason people lose their teeth in the U.S. today.

The best way to prevent gum disease is to practice thorough oral hygiene and have regular professional cleanings. Removing plaque and tartar, which harbor billions of bacteria is the main key with proper nutrition a close second.

Home care has to include daily flossing and brushing at the gum line. Antimicrobial rinses and gum irrigators can help, but are not a substitute for brushing and flossing. Professional dental cleanings are critical as well. People who form tartar quickly and easily are at the greatest risk for gum disease. Since tartar is adhered to the tooth much like a barnacle on a rock, daily brushing will not remove tartar.

People with a history of gum disease or who form tartar easily can benefit from more frequent professional cleanings: every 3-4 months. No more than 6 months should go by between professional cleanings for the rest. During your visits, your gums should be examined for inflammation, and other signs of gum disease. Once a year a full gum measuring (a.k.a. periodontal probing) must be done to keep track of your gum health and identify any areas of acute gum disease.

Although tartar control toothpaste can help reduce tartar formation, many patients find that these toothpastes make their teeth very sensitive. Fortunately, a new home treatment to reduce tartar buildup is now available. ***Therasol Tartar Dissolver*** is an effective and inexpensive product. Although the directions instruct to use it as a rinse, a more effective approach is to "wet brush" with it. Dissolve 1/4 tsp. of the powder in 1 oz. of warm water. Place the liquid in your mouth followed by a toothbrush. A toothbrush with fine bristles that slip better under the gums is ideal. Brush your gums for 2 minutes over a sink incase you drool. Frequency depends on your speed of tartar formation. Have your dentist take a picture of your tartar before a cleaning, then use Therasol Tartar dissolver once a day. At your subsequent cleaning take another photo. Compare the results, evaluate effectiveness and adjust your regimen accordingly.

Vitamin K2, first described by Weston Price as *Factor X* helps to reduce tartar formation as well. Our diet is deficient in vitamin K2 therefore supplementation is advisable. A good choice is Life Extension's Vitamin K2 Complex as it contains both the MK-4 and MK-7 forms.

Excellent home care, regular professional cleanings and gum measuring can be a very effective defense against gum disease.

ORAL HYGIENE

Most plaque and therefore tooth disease gathers at the gum line. This is where you need to focus your efforts. It is common knowledge that good oral home care is important to maintain a disease-free mouth. However, few people know how to do it right. Well today is your lucky day! So pay attention.

Flossing: Most people do not floss. It's hard and time consuming. In adults, most tooth decay and gum disease occurs in between the teeth. So floss only those teeth you want to keep!

Your teeth have 5 cleanable tooth surfaces: the chewing surface, check/lip surface, tongue surface and the 2 side surfaces in between your teeth. Remember, not flossing is like not cleaning $2/5^{th}$ of your teeth. To get in the habit of flossing, do it before you brush. If you leave it for last, you will probably not do it at all.

Brushing: Although electric toothbrushes are very effective, a properly used manual toothbrush is good as well. Only use soft or extra soft bristles. Using a circular motion place the bristles at a 45 degree angle towards your gums and use a press and wiggle motion if using a manual brush or just hold the electric brush in one place. Begin in one place and follow the arch of your mouth all the way around the outside and then the inside returning to where you started. Brush each section for 5 seconds; advance the brush in overlapping segments around all of your teeth. When brushing your back upper teeth, close your mouth half way to create extra room for your toothbrush head.

Tongue cleaning: Your tongue is has thousands of tiny hair like projections called papilla covering its surface. Bacteria, plaque and food particles are often trapped on its surface. Brushing just moves the stuff around, while tongue scraping is very effective. There are may tongue scraper designs. They all act like a squidgy and all are equally effective. The first time you clean your tongue and see what comes off, you will never stop doing it!

Tongue scraping decreases the bacterial volume in your mouth, improves your breath and tongue appearance. Make tongue-scraping part of your daily oral hygiene routine.

Rinses: There are many rinses on the market. Some are anti-bacterial, some have fluoride to help prevent tooth decay, some are all natural, some help prevent tartar and some even whiten your teeth. Using a rinse has to be specific to the individuals needs. Your dentist can help you decide which rinse, if any is good to add to your oral health regimen.

Which is the best toothbrush?

Commercially available toothbrushes come in four varieties: hard, medium, soft and extra soft. Only use soft or extra soft brushes. Medium and hard brushed do not do a better job, they just scratch and injure your teeth and gums and can increase tooth wear. So why are they are sold? Economics: supply and demand, because people buy them. Every year companies come out with new toothbrush head designs. The truth is they are all pretty much the same, so stick with an extra-soft brush if you can find one and change it every 2-3 months and especially after a cold.

Which is the best toothpaste?

Most commercially available toothpastes contain chemicals that are not necessarily good for us. The fact is, toothpaste does not remove plaque and clean your teeth. The cleaning comes from the toothbrush. The function of toothpastes is to remove minor stain and provide topical fluoride. Many types of toothpaste are very abrasive. Different toothpastes may be used to achieve different goals.

Avoid toothpastes with Triclosan. Triclosan is an antibacterial agent that is found in many products, including toothpaste. A major concern with Triclosan is bacterial resistance: the forced evolution of bacterial to resist Triclosan creating a "super bug".

There is some evidence that tooth pastes containing Sodium Laurel Sulfate (SLS) cause canker sores. SLS is a great foaming agent that has been found to cause skin irritations in some people. This surfactant, which is found in industrial cleaners like car wash soaps, shampoos, engine degreasers and floor cleaners, is also found in most popular toothpastes. If you suffer form apthous ulcers, try using toothpastes without SLS. Common brands of toothpaste that do not have SLS include Sensodyne, Sensodyne ProEnamel, Rembrandt G, and Biotene.

Patients who have exposed dentin from erosion, abrasion, attrition or have thin enamel can benefit from Sensodyne ProEnamel which has been shown to thicken enamel and is one of the lowest abrasive tooth pastes on the market.

Many patients suffer from tooth sensitivity. The major cause of tooth sensitivity is exposed dentin tubules. There are two strategies available to reduce tooth sensitivity: make the nerve less sensitive or plug up the open tubules. Potassium Nitrate has been shown to be an effective tooth nerve desensitizer. Most toothpastes for sensitive teeth contain 5%Potsssioum Nitrate. Its effectiveness is dose and time dependent. You must use it twice daily for at least 2-4 weeks to see any effect. Once you stop use, the effects go away. So if Potassium Nitrate containing toothpaste is working for you, keep using it indefinitely. Toothpastes that plug up the dentin tubules include Sensodyne Repair and Protect, MI paste and Renew paste. A good strategy is to start with Sensodyne ProEnamel toothpaste for 1 month, if it is ineffective switch to Sensodyne Repair and Protect.

For those who do not want to use a fluoride containing toothpaste, but are concerned about tooth decay, try using a xylitol containing toothpaste. Look for toothpastes where xylitol is in the first three ingredients listed. An excellent choice is SPRY toothpaste where xylitol is the second ingredient on the list.

Do It Yourself (DIY) Toothpaste.

Many health conscious people use fluoride-free toothpastes that are very expensive. If you want to add topical fluoride to your preventive tooth regimen, use a rinse. Following is a list of ingredients and their function followed by the recipe.

Baking Soda: mild abrasive, safe for enamel, alkaline to combat mouth acids.

Xylitol Powder: antibacterial, helps with calcium absorption of teeth.

Organic Tea Tree Oil: antibacterial.

Organic Oil of Oregano: antibacterial, anti-inflammatory.

Organic Peppermint oil: flavoring.

Organic Unrefined Coconut Oil: antibacterial, nice flavor.

Bentonite Clay: absorbs toxins, heavy metals, and mild abrasive safe for enamel.

These ingredients are easy to find online or at a health food store.

In a glass jar combine 1/4 cup Baking soda, 5 drops tea tree oil, 10 drops Oil of oregano, 15 drops Oil of Peppermint, 1/4 cup organic unrefined coconut oil, 1 tsp. xylitol powder, 1 tsp. Bentonite clay. Mix thoroughly. Place mixture into a zip lock bag, seal and snip off one of the corners with a scissor. Extrude toothpaste mixture into a travel tube available in any drugstore. Use a pea size amount on your toothbrush. Store at room temperature.

UNRAVEL YOUR SMILE FOR BETTER HEALTH

When teeth are misaligned they can be difficult to clean. Gaps and crowding can exacerbate the buildup of bacterial plaque and tartar, making the development of periodontal problems more prevalent. This illustrates the need for straighter teeth—not just for cosmetics, but also more importantly for your health. Misaligned or tipped teeth often are exposed to unhealthy forces causing them to shift, get loose which exacerbates gum disease. To make matters worse, crooked teeth have an increased chance for gum recession and bone loss. Uneven wear and chipping and, root abfractions are another common problem associated with misaligned teeth.

I know what you are thinking: "Braces at my age, no way!" Have no fear, today dentistry has something that may even be better than braces: Invisalign®

Invisalign® is a cosmetic braces alternative, advantages of Invisalign® include:

- It is the most esthetic and cosmetic way to straighten teeth.
- It is made form a Metal-free, BPA-free, FDA approved medical plastic that is a great option for people with metal allergies or metal sensitivities.
- Better gum health because brushing and flossing is easy during treatment.
- Less chance for unsightly white decalcification spots (early cavities) and tooth decay because it is easy to brush and floss during Invisalign® treatment.
- Less need for dental treatment because of decreased incidence of gum disease and tooth decay during treatment.

- Tooth whitening is possible during Invisalign® treatment because the aligners can be used a whitening trays during treatment.
- There is less tooth soreness during treatment
- It is easier to correct cross-bites with Invisalign®.
- The dentist can design your bite in virtual reality.
- There is less injury to lips and cheeks because Invisalign® does not use brackets, wires and braces that can cut the insides of your lips and gums. No need for wax!
- It is easier to eat with Invisalign®. There are no brackets and wires that food will catch on during eating, and no embarrassment during a meal.
- Its removable: if you want to take them off before a date or a business meeting, you can!
- You can see how your teeth will look before you start treatment.
- Less office visits than with braces.

Once Invisalign® treatment is complete, your bite may be improved as well chewing and possibly even your speech. Tooth realignment also relieves stress on the supporting bones and jaw joints, preventing future problems such as gum recession and tooth wear. And of course, your new smile will be straight and beautiful.

Invisalign®, treatment is a 21 century application of an old technique to move teeth. With advanced computer software and aligner production and new innovative features something old has become a better something new. Unlike traditional braces that rely on square metal brackets to pull teeth using wire, Invisalign®, aligners wrap clear, nearly invisible plastic around each tooth to move teeth by gentle pushing and rotating.

With the help of advanced computer technology dentists can create a visual representation of the entire oral arch in 3-D. In this way, fabricated aligners are custom fitted to be worn snugly around the teeth, giving just the right pressure to the misaligned tooth to help lead it back to the desired position. The application of pressure is done in such a way that the brace gently presses on to the teeth. The succeeding series of aligners exerts the right amount of pressure that makes it effective. Replacement of aligner is done every two weeks, with the succeeding series of aligners pre-packed and available to the patient. Most patients need to come in only every 2-3 months for evaluation. Therefore, dental visits are not as frequent as the customary monthly visits required with traditional metal wire braces. This is very convenient for college students or people with busy schedules or who travel.

Invisalign® is constantly improving. Millions are spend on annual research and development. While other companies may make products that look like Invisalign®, they are decades behind in innovation. Recent updates to Invisalign® include a newly redesigned material, SmartTrack. New attachments and tooth movement progression have made Invisalign® a more predictable orthodontic treatment.

TOOTH GRINDING PREVENTION

If one of the questions below is "YES" then you may be a suffering form nighttime tooth grinding or Bruxism.

- Do you suffer from chronic headache, migraines, neck ache or backache?
- Do you wake up with tightness in your jaw or face muscles?
- Do you get clicking or popping in your jaw joint?
- Does your jaw lock in the open or closed position?
- Does your partner complain that you grind your teeth?
- Do you have teeth that are worn or chipped for no apparent reason?
- Do you have sensitive teeth?

- Do you have gum recession root notching or loose teeth?
- Is the lower part of your face becoming shorter or collapsed?
- Are the corners of your mouth always red and irritated?
- Do you have excessive wrinkles around your lips and mouth?

Bruxism is the technical term for harmful clenching and grinding of teeth. People who suffer from bruxism unintentionally bite down too hard at inappropriate times or rub their teeth together. In most cases, it is done while they are sleeping. The fact is that the only time teeth should come together is during swallowing. Any other time this occurs damage to the teeth, muscles of chewing or the Tempero-Mandibular Joint (TMJ) is inevitable. Tooth grinding and clenching is a much more common problem than most people realize. We all grind our teeth to some extent though most of us are not aware of it because the grinding and clenching is done in our sleep. Mild bruxism may not require treatment but moderate to severe bruxism is cumulative and can cause a variety of problems. People with sleep bruxism are often unaware of it until complications develop. Therefore it is important to know the signs and symptoms of teeth grinding and to seek help if you suspect you might have bruxism. (See previous list).

Tooth grinding and clenching is a much more common problem than most people realize. We all grind our teeth to some extent though most of us are not aware of it because the grinding and clenching is done in our sleep. Mild bruxism may not require treatment but moderate to severe bruxism is cumulative and can cause a variety of problems. People with sleep bruxism are often unaware of it until complications develop. Therefore it is important to know the signs and symptoms of teeth grinding and to seek help if you suspect you might have bruxism. (See list above)

The most common treatment is to wear a plastic mouth-guard. These can be bought at a store or made by a dentist. They all serve the same basic function: prevent teeth form coming together and wear prematurely. It is tooth protective only. Unfortunately mouth-guards do not address clenching and may even increase it. Clenching and grinding causes muscle hyperactivity that results in muscle soreness, muscle spasms and muscle pain. Continued clenching and grinding takes a toll on your joints causing arthritis, disc deformation and derangement resulting in pain, clicking, popping, jaw locking in the open or closed position as well as other TMJ problems. In addition, mouth guards are hard to keep clean, build up tartar and can harbor bacteria and yeast. Over time mouth guards get grungy and worn out and need constant replacement depending on your grinding intensity and frequency.

The trouble with mouth-guards: Many people find that wearing mouth-guards at night to be uncomfortable or embarrassing. Often the mouth-guards are spit out during sleep. Most mouth-guards only protect teeth form wear; they do not address the muscles or the TMJ. Mouth-guards are made of plastic, rubber or silicone, which may contain harmful materials such as BPA. In addition, mouth-guards do not address clenching (and may even increase it), muscle hyperactivity (muscle soreness, muscle spasms and muscle pain) and TMJ problems.

Fortunately a new innovative FDA approved device is now available to treat teeth grinding with biofeedback: GRINDCARE. Biofeedback is a well-documented physiological principle using gentle electric impulses to induce local relaxation of specific muscles. Biofeedback is the reason for GRINDCARE's efficient and lasting treatment of teeth grinding or clenching without the need for wearing night-guards. Biofeedback makes your jaws relax. GRINDCARE simply teaches you to stop grinding your teeth. Every time you grind your teeth, the biofeedback device stimulates your jaw muscles with a brief tension impulse, the so-called biofeedback. Biofeedback makes your jaw muscles relax and prevents you from grinding your teeth.

GRINDCARE 3.0 is an innovative wireless device, similar size to an i-pod. The dentist can teach you to use the device so that you can do use it yourself afterwards with ease. All you do is place the small sensor on the chewing muscle of your temple, and then you activate the device following the easy instructions on the screen of the unit. Within less than one minute the treatment has started and will continue while you sleep. In the morning you can see how many times during the night that GRINDCARE has prevented you from grinding or clenching your teeth and creating tension in your jaw muscles. You can see on the screen how successful your treatment is, or in record mode you can see how many times you have been clenching and grinding your teeth.

ORAL CANCER PREVENTION

It is now well established that tobacco use and chronic consumption of alcohol are major risk factors in oral and throat cancer. Elimination tobacco use and curbing alcohol consumption to social events will go along way to reducing your risk of oral cancer.

A less known, but significant risk factor for oral cancer is the human papilloma virus (HPV) infection, the cause of common warts, was found to be a much stronger risk factor than tobacco or alcohol use in a Johns Hopkins University study. Those who had evidence of prior oral HPV infection had a 32-fold increased risk of throat cancer. In addition HPV16, one of the most common cancer-causing strains of the virus, was present in the tumors of 72% of cancer patients in the study. A vaccine, which protects against cervical cancer caused by HPV strains 6, 11, 16 and 18, and also against genital warts, is available. Mouth warts are not uncommon findings in careful dental examinations. Make sure your dentist performs a thorough oral cancer examination at every check up exam. Today, oral warts are can be easily removed with lasers, which eliminates bleeding and stitches

Green Tea: A New Weapon For Oral Cancer Prevention

According to researchers at the University of Texas MD Anderson cancer center, green tea extract may provide a vital role in oral cancer prevention in patients with pre-malignant white patch condition known as oral leukoplakia. The study found that half of the patients who took the green tea extract three times per day over the course of three months had a positive response without any significant side effects. These findings are encouraging for oral cancer patients.

FOR FUTURE MOTHERS

If you are considering starting a family you may want to seriously consider replacing your mercury fillings. Mercury is highly toxic. The most dangerous form of mercury is mercury vapor as it is easily ionized. Ionized mercury vapor can easily pass and invade our body as well as the fetus. Every time you chew, consume hot food or beverages or grind your teeth, mercury vapor escapes form you amalgam mercury-silver fillings. Exposing your developing baby to toxic mercury can lead to miscarriage, birth defects, lower IQ, and preterm birth. Replacing your mercury fillings before you begin conception may be a wise choice for your future children as well as your own health.

DENTISTRY DURING PREGNANCY

It is common for women avoid dental care during pregnancy. The result is that small dental problems can turn into large and expensive ones. Since most mothers refrain from going to the dentist for several months and even years after giving birth as they are caught up in caring for their new infant, they may become victims of unintentional dental neglect.

Fortunately, newer scientific evidence has shed more light on the safety of dental treatment of pregnant women. Research indicates that mothers who receive dental care through the second trimester, both restorative dental care and gum disease treatment, do not appear to increase risk of adverse events during pregnancy. A recent study reported that pregnant women, most with early to moderate periodontitis, benefitted from general and periodontal care without an increase in preterm births or other negative pregnancy outcomes. Another study found a slight association between improvement in a mother's gum health and higher cognitive and motor skills in their children.

Caution should be exercised during the first trimester; dental treatment should be limited to emergency dental treatment. The first trimester is dominated by development of tissues and organs, which may be effected by the administration of medicines during dental care. While the second and third trimesters are devoted to growth. In light of the new research, going the dentist during the second and third trimesters is considered safe.

It may be prudent seek out a dentist who does not use toxic materials in the office. This is critical for dental treatment during pregnancy. Find a dentist who is mercury free, BPA-free. Air filters, UV air cleansers and air ionizers should be used during dental treatment to create a safer atmosphere. Dental lasers for cavity treatment will eliminate or minimize the patients need for local anesthetics. Although x-rays are not usually taken during pregnancy, sometimes in emergency situations it may become necessary. Use of a double-shielded aprons and digital x-rays are used that emit over 90% less radiation than traditional x-rays is advisable. Great care and thought must be made to ensure the safety of your baby.

Monkey See . . .

Studies show that children are more likely to visit the dentist as adults if their parents do. Whether or not children receive regular dental care is strongly associated with their parents' history of seeking dental. At a time when consumption of refined carbohydrates is on rise paralleled by the increase of tooth decay, child obesity and diabetes it is time for parents to closely examine how their behavior and heath habits affect their children.

In addition, a new study confirmed the linkage between parents and children when it came to dental phobia and dental anxiety. High levels of dental fear in the parents are transmitted to the children. Fathers played the biggest role in the transmission of fear.

Healthy Body

The health of your body affects the health of your mouth. Studies show that obesity increases your risk of gum disease, tooth decay and cancer. A poor immune system and body inflammation predisposes you to more infection, including gum disease and tooth decay. A healthy diet and exercise regimen will go a long way to improve the health of your mouth.

NUTRITIOUS DIET

The Standard American Diet (SAD) is very poor in nutrition. In contrast our ancestral diet was rich in good fats, proteins and limited in carbohydrates and rich in antioxidants and phytochemicals. Proper nutrition is critical for supporting our immune system and providing the building blocks for the repair of our body. Vegetables contain a dense collection of hundreds of vitamins, minerals, antioxidants and phytochemicals critical for optimal function.

Some basic dietary guidelines:

* Do not eat processed, human-made or human-altered food.
* Consume a diet rich in leafy greens: make a "Jumbo Salad" or a Green Smoothie.

* Supplement with a good quality Fish or Krill oil and eat plenty of small fish like sardines and shellfish.
* Eat plenty of sea vegetables and seaweed or add a dash of Main Coast Organic Seaweed Flakes to your meals for your natural iodine source.
* Supplement with magnesium, selenium and vitamin K2
* Eliminate all grains, sugar, legumes and dairy (except butter and some cheeses)
* Eat grass-fed/pastured or wild meat, poultry and fish.
* Eat Omega 3 or pastured eggs.
* Take a good quality probiotic: refrigerated is best.

In addition,

* Get 7-9 hours of sleep in a dark room.
* Reduce light exposure after dark.
* 1-2 hours of low intensity exercise (walking, swimming, biking, kayaking, stand up paddle boarding): 2-3 days a week.
* 1 day of interval sprinting 20 min.
* 1-2 days of high intensity training: lifting weights (30 min)

Dr. Shvartsman's Green Smoothie:

Variety is key. While juicing concentrates nutrients, it also concentrates sugar and removes fiber. Fiber is critical to slow down sugar absorption. Remember, in nature the higher the sugar, the higher the fiber: sugar cane is high in sugar and it's a stick! A great way to get your fiber and nutrients at the same time is by using a high-powered blender like the Nutri Bullet.

Recommended ingredients:

½ cup Kale or other greens, ½ cup spinach, ½ cup bokchoy, 1 carrot, ½ avocado, 1 tsp. fresh ginger, 1 clove garlic, ½ green apple, 1 tbsp. organic unrefined coconut oil ½ cup coconut water, ¼ tsp. ground turmeric, ¼ tsp. ground cinnamon.

TOOTH DECAY

Tooth Decay is a bacterial infiltration of the tooth. Much like an infection. Dentally known as **caries**, tooth decay is a Neolithic disease. Prior to agriculture, tooth decay was non-existent. No other animal on earth gets tooth decay. Actually that's not true, our pets get tooth decay too. Ever wonder why???

Our hunter-gatherer ancestors did not have tooth decay, their skulls prove that. Tooth Decay is a man-made disease. Civilization and convenience, along with population growth have led to our processed-food diet. The Standard American Diet (SAD) is high in carbs, sugar, toxins, nutrient binding chemicals and is mostly devoid of key nutrients necessary for optimal health and well-being.

Tooth decay significantly weakens teeth. It unravels their intricate structure, destroying the key support element in our chewing apparatus a.k.a. our *masticatory system*. Most synthetic tooth restorative materials are so different from the natural tooth structure that the tooth further breaks, sometimes beyond the possibility of restoration. Tooth decay is second only to gum disease in the leading reason why people loose their teeth, today. Fortunately, now exist a number of dental restorative materials that mimic the physical properties of the tooth. You just have to know what to look for . . .

How to "heal a cavity"

Studies conducted in the 1960's showed that softened enamel could be completely healed with remineralizing dental treatment. This natural process of *re-mineralization* makes the softened enamel strong again by replacing the lost minerals within the enamel. Pushing a sharp pointy metal pick into a weakened area of the tooth reduced the chance of such repair. Natural enamel can rebuild itself and heal a soft spot. This occurs rapidly if the enamel surface remains intact. The repair process becomes more complicated or even impossible if the surface is broken.

The fact is that cavity detection with the explorer picking technique is not very effective in detecting cavities when they start. A study published in 1992 showed that the explorer technique based on finding "sticky spots" was only 24% accurate in finding true dental decay in pits and groves of the teeth. At best, other studies showed up to 64% accuracy. This is because the sharp point can be wedged in a perfectly healthy pit or groove giving the dentist a sticky feel even if there is not decay at all! In addition, many teeth have stained grooves and pits that are not decay. So they appear to be cavities. Stain can be mistaken for tooth decay. It is probable that many teeth have been needlessly drilled and filled for this reason.

Even more troubling is that many early or small cavities go untreated because the dentist does not always feel a stick. Meanwhile, the enamel has begun to lose its minerals in the process of de-mineralization, the first stage in tooth decay. This is common with white or brown spots on teeth. When these early cavities are left untreated they will process into the deeper layer of the tooth and become large cavities that need removing. This can lead to unnecessary fillings, root canal treatment, crowns or extractions.

White spots on enamel or rough areas of the tooth can be a sign of the beginning of a cavity. Blunted or dulled explorers should be used to feel the enamel and never pushed forcibly on the tooth.

One of the greatest advances in tooth decay diagnosis has been the Laser Cavity Scanner called the Diagnodent. This laser is over 90% effective in **painlessly** finding event the smallest cavities early. This Laser gives an indication of bacterial levels in pits and grooves of the tooth as well as any smooth area on the tooth. The instrument gives a numerical read out that both the patient and the dentist can see. It's like having a second opinion that is better then the old fashioned "stick the sharp pointy metal pick into a tooth" method. Many phobic or dentally anxious patients really appreciate this accurate and pain free and anxiety reducing modern instrument.

REVERSING TOOTH DECAY

Our saliva has a natural cavity reversing mechanism. Unfortunately, tooth decay is on the rise Globally and in the U.S. due to increased consumption of processed and refined carbohydrates and sugar. Several products are available to help strengthen teeth and reduce tooth decay rates. It is possible to reverse early enamel cavities and prevent new cavities from forming through the natural process of re-mineralization. Newly available products containing Amorphous Calcium Phosphate (ACP) are very effective in improving re-mineralization by supplying a readily available source of Calcium and Phosphate, the building blocks to enamel, Along with Xylitol and topically applied Fluoride tooth decay can be addressed through 3 different yet synergistic mechanisms. This non-invasive, drill-free protocol is a powerful tool to help people prone to tooth decay.

DRILL-FREE FILLINGS

White spots on your teeth are the result of weakened, demineralized enamel. They are often the first sign of the start of a cavity. Many patients find these white spots unsightly. ICON represents an entirely new, revolutionary approach to treatment of incipient cavities—a resin infiltrate. ICON can cosmetically remove white spots in just one visit! This provides a highly esthetic alternative to destructive treatments of white spots—all in one simple treatment, with no drilling, no shots, no noise and in just 10 minutes per tooth!

ICON treatment enables dentists to immediately treat cavities not yet advanced enough for conventional restoration and ends the "watch and wait" approach. It stops tooth decay progress without unnecessary loss of healthy tooth structure. ICON allows for a conservative cosmetic treatment of small cavities. Patients with poor compliance to re-mineralization protocols are excellent candidates. ICON is not just minimally invasive dentistry . . . it is micro-invasive.

The ICON process: The tooth is cleaned, and treated with an acid to open up the enamel and dentin. The tooth is then dried with alcohol. Utilizing a specially developed infuser tip an ultra thin resin is applied to the tooth surface. Through capillary action, similar to a sponge soaking up water, the weakened enamel and dentin absorb an ultra thin resin over a period of 3 minutes. The tooth surface is then wiped clean and the resin is hardened with a specialized blue LED light. That's it! You can go have lunch, meet with a client or simply enjoy not being numb for several hours.

When the decay has progressed past the enamel into the dentin it is not possible to reverse the decay. Mechanical removal of the cavity is necessary to stop the progression of the cavity. If caught early enough, modern dentistry has provided dentists with a drill free solution: The Laser. Dentists can virtually painlessly vaporize the decay and bacteria using an Er:Yag dental laser. It cleans out the cavity and sterilizes the area helping to prevent further tooth decay under the filling.

MODERN ADVANCES IN TOOTH DECAY REMOVAL

In the early 1800's dentists were taught to drill out all non-decayed grooves and pits in teeth and fill them with amalgam of silver and mercury to prevent cavities in a process called "extension for prevention". This resulted in unnecessary weakening of teeth and a lot more mercury in people's mouth. This practice is still taught in every dental school in the USA.

There are two types of decay deep inside the tooth: Infected and Affected dentin. Infected dentin is full of bacteria and has to be thoroughly removed, otherwise the cavity will continue to progress, affected dentin is softer than healthy dentin, but it can be left and when a properly sealed filling is placed it will re-mineralize and become hard again. The trouble is, it is impossible to tell which is which. This is a problem when the cavity is very deep and close to the nerve. Fortunately, several new technologies are now available to help dentists remove only the bacteria infected part of the tooth.

It is now possible to stain infected dentin. The stain was developed in Japan in 1978. This way the dentist knows exactly where the healthy and the diseased part of the tooth are. The old fashioned approach to pick at the tooth to identify decay is fraught with error and when the decay is very close to the nerve it is possible to poke through the thin dentin into the nerve!

Once the decay is identified with the dye, dentists can use a newly developed line of ceramic and resin burs to selectively remove infected dentin and leave the healthy tooth intact. A laser decay scanner called the Diagnodent can further be used to verify that all the infected dentin has been removed. A numerical read out correlated to histologically verified infected or affected dentin.

Ozone is a great disinfectant. It selectively destroys bacteria yeast and fungus, yet is completely safe to humans. However there are two problems with its use: it is not FDA approved for dental use and it reduces the bond strength of the filling to the tooth by approximately 50%. This makes it not very useful when a bonded resin-composite filling is used to restore the tooth.

Air-Abrasion is another useful device used to clean out cavities without a drill. As stream of fine medical grade porcelain powder is used to "sand blast" away tooth decay. Newer devices add a water jet to minimize dust formation from the powder. It is reported that most small to medium cavities can be cleaned out without the need to numb the patient. This technology gives similar resutst to the Er:Yag laser.

TOOH CONSERVING DENTISTRY: A MODERN PARADIGM

The fact is: ***there is no synthetic material as good as your own natural tooth structure.*** Unfortunately, traditional dental techniques for restoring teeth are relatively aggressive and tooth destructive to the modern techniques. Most dentists are still using mercury-amalgam fillings and crowns to rebuild teeth. These techniques were developed in the 1800s and changed very little in the past few centuries. However, the last 3 decades have brought us a whirlwind of dental advances in both materials and technology and with them as new approach—Tooth Conserving Dentistry—to restoring weakened teeth without destroying more healthy tooth structure.

Mercury-amalgam fillings were designed in the early 1800's. The material is a mainly equal parts of silver powder and liquid mercury, with some tin, copper and a few other trace metals. Although many patients are worried about the health effects of mercury in their fillings, what they may not know is how tooth destructive amalgam fillings really are.

Once all of the decay is cleaned out of the tooth, dentists are taught to further drill away healthy tooth structure from any grooves and pits in the tooth, even though there is no further decay present. This is called "extension for prevention". Unfortunately this approach further weakens an already decay-compromised tooth. Since mercury amalgam fillings are brittle when thin, dentists who place mercury-amalgam fillings have to drill deeper into the tooth when there is a only a shallow cavity in order to achieve the minimum mercury-amalgam thickness. In addition, because mercury-amalgam fillings are not bonded to the tooth, dentists have to place undercuts in the tooth to keep the filling from falling out. This is based on wood working techniques where the base has to be wider than the top, also known as a "dove tail joint". Often retentive grooves and pits are used as well. All these methods require additional drilling away of perfectly healthy tooth structure, which further weakens the tooth and makes it more prone to fracture. Another mercury-amalgam retention technique is placing small pins into tooth. These pins can cause micro cracks, and can accidentally puncture into the nerve or out of the side of the tooth requiring root canal treatment or tooth extraction. As if this was not bad enough, since mercury-amalgam fillings are so different from the physical properties of the tooth such as expansion and contraction with heat and cold, flexure, and compression, cracks can and do develop from the inside out. At best these cracks cause the tooth to break above the gum, but sometimes the tooth can split in half like a log and has to be extracted. Even small metal fillings can split teeth in half.

When the tooth is damaged beyond the point when a filling can be placed a stronger restoration is indicated. Most dentists use crowns for this purpose. Crowns that require drilling the tooth down to a nub or a stump. Often strong, healthy parts of the tooth are drilled away and are flushed down the drain. Once healthy tooth structure is removed it is gone forever. This can further weaken a tooth and traumatize the nerve leading to nerve death, pain and the need for root canal treatment.

Today, tooth-conserving restorations can be used in place of full crowns to restore only the weak or damaged parts of the tooth.

BIOMIMETIC DENTISTRY

"When it comes to biology, nature is and will always be better than anything man will ever invent."

Dr. Alex Shvartsman

The further we displace ourselves from our natural way of being the worse it is for our body and health. This is an undeniable and profound truth.

The importance of respecting nature has recently been exemplified in studies of human jaw development. One study has found that children who are breast-fed develop properly shaped upper jaws as opposed to those who are artificially fed with a typical narrow bottle. Another important point when it comes to breastfeeding is that what nature has designed for babies to eat will always be far superior to any man-made formula. Another study found that children in hunter-gatherer groups, eating unprocessed food develop normal lower jaws as opposed to children eating a mushy highly pureed processed food diet we feed our babies today. Eating natural food that is our birthright not only is good for our health it is critical for our jaw development. It is no wonder that most children in the US need braces because their jaws are too small to accommodate their teeth.

Our hunter-gatherer ancestors had straight teeth and an absence of tooth decay and gum disease. For hundreds of thousands of years before agriculture, which is only 10-5 thousand years old, human beings lived one with nature as hunter-gatherers eating a diet of animals, vegetables and fruit. Grains, legumes and dairy were not part of their natural diet, no matter which environment they lived in. It is only with the advent of grain, legume and dairy and sugar consumption do we find tooth decay and gum disease. This is something to consider if you want to avoid these common diseases of the mouth in our westernized society.

When it comes to restoring teeth, dentists also need to look to nature as the blue print. This is why the direction dentistry must follow is a biomimetic approach to restring decayed and weakened teeth. Biomimetic Dentistry focuses on restoring teeth with materials that closely emulate the different parts of the tooth in physical structure, esthetic form and color. By respecting what is natural biomimetic dentists always take great care to preserve as much of the natural tooth as possible. By using materials that replicate the physics of the tooth, fillings, partial crowns veneers and crowns will work in harmony with the tooth and not against it.

Our teeth are a remarkable feat of biologic engineering. In fact, human teeth are designed so well that they have not changed for the past 250,000 years. Their perfect design is a balance between biologic, mechanical, functional, and esthetic parameters.

Biomimetics can be defined as "the study of structure and function of biological systems as models for the design and engineering of materials". "Biomimetic Dentistry", a term coined by Dr. Pascal Magne, a professor at the University of Southern California is defined as the reconstruction of teeth to emulate their natural biomechanical an esthetic form and function. Biomimetic Dentistry is the most current, science-supported approach to treating weak, fractured, and decayed teeth in a way that keeps them strong and seals them from bacterial invasion. Biomimetic Dentistry has the potential to make restored teeth last significantly longer.

Dentists that follow this approach, focus on reproducing the biomechanics and esthetic properties of intact healthy teeth using the latest techniques and materials. Biomimetic dentists study and strive to fully understand the stress and strain of individual teeth under function. This allows restorative techniques to be optimized and the right materials to be used to rebuild the various layers of your teeth. Unfortunately, most dentists are still using antiquated Civil War age fillings and crowns in a world of space age materials and techniques.

Careful sealing against infection eliminates the need for 60% to 90% of the crowns and root canal treatments of traditional "drill and fill" dentistry. Biomimetic dentists do not simply "dig out decay and fill holes". They restore teeth using modern adhesive materials, composite fillings and porcelains in a way that rebuilds teeth as close to their original structure, function and esthetics as possible with today's most current dental materials. The underlying principle of Biomimetic Dentistry is tooth conservative dentistry. Every effort is made to conserve as much of your own healthy teeth as possible.

Recently a team of dentists, including Dr. Alex Shvartsman, formed the Academy of Biomimetic Dentistry. The purpose of this nonprofit organization of biomimetic dentists is to of educate other dentists in the philosophy and techniques of Biomimetic Dentistry so that more patients may benefit from healthier, longer lasting dental restorations. There are currently only about 220 Biomimetic Dentists in the United States.

Unfortunately there is much resistance in the dental community to these ideas. Therefore, people need to take charge of their health and become their own health care advocates. As public demand for healthier dentistry grows, perhaps Biomimetic Dentistry will become the norm and not the exception in how teeth are restored in the future.

AMALGAM FILLINGS

IS THERE POISON IN YOUR TEETH?

Amalgam fillings were first invented in 1819 as a cheap substitute to cemented gold fillings and crowns. At the time they were the only direct teeth filling material available to dentists. Amalgam fillings are made up of roughly 55% mercury and 45% metal powder containing mostly silver with traces of zinc, and tin and copper. When combined together this metal mixture slowly solidifies into a hard metal amalgam. Although the fillings look like a metal alloy, in fact all the metals are separate, including mercury. Once packed into the tooth, the metal amalgam then begins to corrode. This corrosion is looked at favorably as it apparently forms a seal between the tooth and the filling. Besides filling in the gap between the tooth and the filling, the amalgam corrosive rust constantly leaches into the mouth.

Mercury is the only metal that is in liquid form at room temperature. It readily vaporizes from its liquid state into a colorless, odorless, tasteless gas. It is an extraordinarily powerful poison. In fact, mercury is the most poisonous naturally occurring non-radioactive substance on earth. It is toxic in micrograms (mcg), while other heavy metals such as cadmium, lead and arsenic are toxic in milligrams making mercury 100 times more toxic. One microgram of mercury vapor contains 3 trillion atoms of mercury. There are no safe levels of mercury.

In 1979, a University of Iowa study reported a measurable release of mercury vapor from amalgam fillings. Vapor release became much greater during chewing, brushing or exposure to hot or acidic foods. These findings were later confirmed in 1981 by an Ohio State University study. Despite these findings both the ADA and the NIH claim there are no harmful health effects from mercury in amalgam fillings and condone its use.

The amount of mercury vapor released from mercury fillings is directly proportional to the temperature the filling is exposed to. Any stimulation of amalgam fillings releases mercury vapor. More mercury vapor is released from high copper amalgam fillings, which are popular today.

Tests using the Jerome mercury vapor analyzer, which is an industry standard in detection mercury vapor showed the following results: Chewing releases 40 micrograms of mercury per cubic meter (mcg/ m3), brushing releases 200 mcg/Hg/m3, tooth grinding releases 350 mcg/Hg/m3, polishing during a cleaning releases 600 mcg/Hg/m3 and unsafe removal is over 1000 mcg/Hg/m3, which is the limit of the Jerome mercury vapor analyzer.

After decades of resistance, the American Food and Drug Administration (FDA) finally supported the phase-out of mercury containing amalgam fillings for a select portion of the population. In June 2008, the FDA conceded after settling a lawsuit with several consumer advocacy groups that amalgam fillings containing mercury may cause health problems with pregnant women, children and fetuses. As part of the settlement, the FDA agreed to alert consumers about potential risks on its website. That warning was subsequently taken off without any explanation to the public.

In 2009 a bill endorsed by 19 members of Congress was written to ban mercury amalgam use in children and pregnant women due to health concerns. This bill was rejected by the Obama administration days before the bill was to become law. Many believe this was not a health oriented, but a politically oriented decision to maintain cheaper dental care as a precursor to the Socialized Government Health Care initiative. In contrast, Denmark, Norway, Sweden, Scandinavia and Finland have banned the use of mercury amalgam fillings.

A poll of 2,590 U.S. adults conducted in 2006, found that 72% of respondents were not aware that mercury was a main component of dental amalgam, and 92% of respondents would prefer to be told about mercury in dental amalgam before receiving it as a filling. This could be compared to being given a drug today by a pharmacy without the mandated FDA prescribing information. In California dentists are required by law to hang signs in their reception areas informing patients about the mercury content of "silver" fillings. Sadly, in other states, many dentists continue to place mercury-containing fillings without informing their patients of dental amalgam fillings' its mercury content.

A 2011 American Dental Association (ADA) survey found that dental amalgam is used as the major tooth filling material. In the U.S. the highest usage is in the Pacific Northwest and lowest in Florida.

Finally, after years of denial about the toxicity of amalgam fillings, the United States government has announced its support of a "phase down" of mercury amalgam fillings. Now the U.S. government endorses the protection children and the unborn from amalgam and recommended that a global educational effort be made to protect children and fetuses.

Finally, a recent study had unequivocally demonstrated a connection to health problems and mercury fillings. In 1998, in a study was commissioned by the a leading dental organization, where a group of Portuguese orphans were followed for 10 years from the ages of 8 to 18. Half were treated with mercury fillings, the other half with composite resin fillings. Not surprisingly, the evaluation of the data showed no relationship.

However, when an independent group of scientists looked at the data and plotted it correctly, the results were disturbing. This re-analysis was driven by the Geier team, which has published a number of studies on both mercury and autism. They re-analyzed the Portugal data into four data points (high, medium low, and no amalgam), instead of the original two, thus allowing the dose-response trend to be finally observable. The 2011 Geier publication prompted the original team (Woods et al, at the University of Washington) to reanalyze the data and confirm the harm from mercury fillings.

Sadly, none of this was reported in any dental journal.

MERCURY TOXISITY

The most dangerous form of mercury is mercury vapor, the kind that is emitted by mercury fillings when they are stimulated by chewing or hot foods and beverages. Mercury vapor is easily ionized. It is the ionic form of mercury gas that easily penetrates our cells and causes significant damage. The negative health effects of chronic mercury exposure on the body is cumulative and can take decades to manifest. Mercury affects our immune system and depletes the body of powerful antioxidants such as glutathione.

Chronic mercury toxicity can result in neurologic impairment leading emotional and mental effects which include to fits of anger, anxiety, apathy, confusion, depression, fear, lack of concentration, lethargy, memory loss, mood swings, nervousness, stuttering and speech impairment and suicide. In fact, dentists have the highest rate of suicide than any other profession. Students are never taught in dental school that their future careers may be a health hazard. Mercury directly or indirectly makes other diseases worse.

Besides the brain, the kidneys and lungs are also greatly affected. Chronic mercury poisoning is also related to allergies, anemia asthma, chest pain, chronic tiredness, tremors, chronic coughing, hair loss, headaches, join and muscle aches, irregular heartbeat, tinnitus (ringing in the ears), sore throat, and vision problems. While other causes for these conditions and symptoms exist, there is no way to determine how the degree mercury toxicity has contributed to these symptoms.

Mercury poisoning can result in several diseases, including acrodynia (pink disease), Hunter-Russell syndrome, and Minamata disease and Fanconi syndrome and can contribute or exacerbate ALS, Alzimers, arthritis, candidiasis, chronic fatigue syndrome, dementia, diabetes, fibromyalgia, Multiple sclerosis, Parkinson's disease, and thyroid disease.

Common physical symptoms of mercury poisoning include nerve damage presenting as numbness, itching, burning, tingling or pain in fingers or toes. Skin discoloration: pink cheeks, fingertips and toes as well as swelling, peeling or shedding of skin. A person suffering from mercury poisoning may experience profuse sweating, persistently faster-than-normal heartbeat, increased salivation, and high blood pressure. Affected children may show red cheeks nose and lips, loss of hair, teeth and nails. Transient rashes, muscle weakness, and increased sensitivity to light are common. Other symptoms may include memory impairment, insomnia, and emotional problems. If you are experiencing any of these symptoms and have a mouth full of mercury fillings, you may want to consider removing them and having mercury toxicity testing and read the rest of this chapter.

If you are planning a family, consider the fact that ionized mercury vapor from the mother's mercury fillings can easily penetrate the cells in not only her body, but her developing child as well. Exposure to the unborn child can begin as early as conception, continues through fetal development and throughout nursing. Fetal exposure to mercury can result in spontaneous abortion, stillbirth, congenital malformations, infertility, learning and developmental disorders, low birth weight and autism.

In a 2013 statement, the IAOMT had the following to say regarding a recent ADA statement that mercury amalgam fillings are safe:

"The International Academy of Oral Medicine and Toxicology (IAOMT) vehemently disputes recent allegations made by the American Dental Association (ADA) that there is no scientific evidence validating the harmful health effects of dental mercury fillings.

James M. Love, J.D., legal counsel to the IAOMT, responded, "The ADA continues to support its self-serving view by denying that mercury fillings are dangerous. Clearly, public health is not an ADA priority."

Silver-colored dental amalgam fillings contain 55% mercury, a known neurotoxin, and the ADA's latest defense of these fillings came as a retort to a March 28th segment on The Dr. Oz Show entitled "Are Your Silver Fillings Making Your Sick?" Dr. Oz, dentists, and other guests warned viewers about dangers of dental mercury.

The following day, the ADA issued a press release accusing Dr. Oz of "sensationalism" and declaring that "not one credible scientific study" shows dental mercury is a health risk.

Contrary to ADA's position, the IAOMT has catalogued hundreds of scientific studies dating back over a century demonstrating that mercury in dental fillings is hazardous to human health. In fact, in 1845, the American Society of Dental Surgeons, the ADA's predecessor, required its members to pledge not to use mercury containing dental amalgam fillings because mercury was known to be extremely toxic, yet in 1859 the ADA was founded based on its endorsement of these controversial fillings.

In more recent years, Norway, Sweden, and Denmark have banned the use of mercury fillings, and other countries have restricted their use for pregnant women, children, and patients with kidney problems, including the US FDA.

In 1991 and 2003, the World Health Organization (WHO) confirmed that dental amalgam is the greatest source of human exposure to mercury in the general population, and in 2005, a WHO report listed adverse health effects caused by mercury exposure, cautioning, "Recent studies suggest that mercury may have no threshold below which some adverse effects do not occur." Meaning that there is **NO SAFE LEVELS OF MERCURY.**

On its dental amalgam webpage in 2008, the United States Food and Drug Administration (FDA) warned about dental mercury's potential neurotoxic effects on children and fetuses, but later removed the warning without explanation.

Later, at a 2010 FDA Dental Products Panel meeting to discuss the health impacts of mercury amalgam fillings, Dr. Suresh Kotagal, a pediatric neurologist at the Mayo Clinic, concluded, " . . . I think that there is really no place for mercury in children."

The same FDA Panel encouraged consideration for limiting dental mercury for pregnant women and children, as well as labeling to warn consumers of the mercury risks. The public was told that FDA's ruling on the issue would be made by December 31, 2011. However, no action has been taken to date.

Amalgam risk assessments conducted in 1995, 2010, and 2012 by Dr. G. Mark Richardson, an expert to the European Union's Scientific Committee on Health and Environmental Risks (SCHER), revealed that toxic levels of mercury were released from dental fillings. Other risk assessments confirm these findings.

Additional "credible" scientific research released in 2012 includes a Yale University study substantiating occupational dental mercury exposure, two studies corroborating the harmful impacts of mercury fillings on children and adolescents, and a study demonstrating that maternal amalgam fillings release mercury into breast milk.

Opponents to the ADA's position on mercury fillings cite a 1995 legal brief filed by ADA attorneys asserting, "The ADA owes no legal duty of care to protect the public from allegedly dangerous products used by dentists. The ADA did not manufacture, design, supply or install the mercury-containing amalgams."

Similarly, last year, the ADA lobbied the U.S. Department of State to oppose a ban or limit on the use of amalgam fillings in connection with the United Nations Environment Programme's legally-binding mercury treaty. However, the treaty text agreed upon in January includes the global phase-down of dental mercury fillings.

Dr. William Virtue, DDS, President of the IAOMT, is concerned. "While worldwide action is being taken to protect humans and the environment from mercury, the ADA continues to mislead the public into believing that one of the most toxic elements on this planet somehow becomes less poisonous when it is placed in their mouths."

MERCURY TOXISITY TESTING

While there are many direct tests for mercury, they are ineffective to assess the mercury bound within cells or organs in your body. Mercury toxicity is best measured indirectly by studying the effects of mercury on our body. One of the simplest a most telling tests is the **fractionated urine porphoryn** test. Of all the body organs, the kidneys harbor the most mercury, especially if the exposure is chronic over many years as occurs with mercury fillings.

Mercury uniquely disrupts 3 key enzymes in the *heme* pathway, causing a buildup of porphoryns. Obtaining a fractionated urine porphoryn assay is therefore very telling of mercury toxicity to the kidney. In addition, this test is very effective in evaluating kidney health.

Any major lab can run this test. It is critical to follow strict collection protocol in order to obtain the best sample. Make sure you are given a dark jar, as light will disrupt the sample. Collect your first urine of the day in a darkened room. This is best done at home. You lab will provide you with the appropriate sample container. Most doctors will not be aware of this test because it is seldom used. Seek out a holistic physician or open-minded doctor. If a dentist orders this test you may not get insurance coverage.

First Mercury toxicity gene identified!

As much as we are all about the same, each of us is individually different. Our genes and our environment each paly a role. For the first time a gene has been identified that may shine some light on why some people are more susceptible to mercury than others. The re-analysis of the Portugal Children's Amalgam Trial now shows that boys with a common genetic variant of the CPOX4 gene incurred the greatest harm from mercury amalgam fillings. This finding validates the genetic-susceptibility theory of dental amalgam. While a genetic test for the CPOX4 gene is not currently available, concerned people who feel that mercury from their amalgam fillings is negatively impacting their health can choose to have their amalgam fillings safely removed by a well trained dentist.

METAL AMALGAM FILLINGS MAY BE DANGEROUS FOR YOUR TEETH

The majority of American dentists use amalgam fillings. Dental amalgam is the most popular filling material sold in the USA today. Aside from the health concerns of mercury fillings, there still is another major concern that is largely never discussed: the potential direct damage to teeth from amalgam fillings.

Amalgam fillings are not cemented in to the tooth like an inlay or a crown. The only technology available in the 1800's to keep amalgam fillings in place were basic wood working principles. These include a dovetail joint design: the base needed to be wider than the top so the filling would not fall out of the tooth. Since a cavity creates a bowl shaped hole, the undercutting of healthy tooth to hold the fillings in place is necessary. For replacing huge fillings, cusp holes are drilled and pins are screwed into the tooth; this can lead to micro crack formation, tooth perforation and even nerve trauma, which can lead root canal treatment or tooth extraction.

Not only do mercury fillings do nothing to rebuilding the integrity of the tooth following decay removal, they additionally further weaken the tooth by requiring the removal of additional healthy tooth structure. To make matters worse, silver-mercury fillings expand with time and heat putting pressure on the already compromised tooth. This can have dire consequences: catastrophic tooth fracture.

Proponents of amalgam fillings praise the fillings' longevity. Some amalgam fillings can last decades. While this is true, the bigger question is, "At what cost to the tooth?" If that cost is a weakened tooth that cracks, breaks or splits in half and needs extraction, then perhaps that risk is too great, especially when better alternatives exist today.

Fortunately there is an alternative to silver-mercury amalgam fillings. Since the 1980's bonded, tooth colored, resin composite fillings have evolved into predictable, long lasting restorations.

SAFER MERCURY FILLING REMOVAL

Many people are concerned about the health ramifications of having their mercury containing amalgam fillings replaced. They understand that care needs to be taken to minimize their exposure to toxic mercury vapor during amalgam filling removal. Silver-mercury amalgam fillings consist of combined metals, including silver, zinc, mercury, tin and copper. These fillings contain about 55% mercury, the most toxic nonradioactive elements on earth.

Since amalgam fillings contain mercury, properly trained dentists do everything possible to reduce their patient's exposure to mercury vapor during amalgam removal. The International Academy of Oral Medicine and Toxicology (IAOMT) has established a protocol (also known as the Huggins protocol) to help minimize people's exposure to mercury. As a concerned patient one should know the basics of the protocol. Although membership in the IAOMT does not guarantee the dentist adheres to the protocol, accredited members of the IAOMT (AIAOMT) pass a written and oral test on dental toxicology and safe mercury removal protocol outlined next.

The Process

The teeth are isolated with a rubber dam so that no amalgam pieces and debris enter the mouth. It is important that the rubber dam is latex free (nitrile) as latex is permeable to mercury vapor. A nose mask attached to 100% oxygen is used to protect the patient from inhaling the highly ionizable mercury vapor, which is generated in high amounts during drilling. The amalgam filling is sectioned in large chunks in order to minimizing the pulverization (drilling) of the amalgam and thus reducing the vaporization of the mercury. Copious amounts of water are used to cool the drill and amalgam dust thereby reducing the vaporization of the mercury. The high-speed suction is placed next to the filling being removed to remove the water, amalgam particles, mercury and to suction off the mercury vapor. A saliva ejector is placed under the rubber dam next to the area where the filling is being removed. This is done as a form of protection to suction any vapor that may escape under the rubber dam. Following the procedure the mouth is rinsed and any amalgam dust and particles are suctioned out. Every patient should wear eye protection for their safety as well as a full body drape.

Each treatment room should be equipped with a tri-functional air purifier device. Which has an independent HEPA air filtration system to remove airborne particles. The air ionizer is important to remove the mercury and other heavy metal particles that have escaped into the room and the UV system, which kills any airborne bacteria and viruses. Each patient is covered with a full torso drape to minimize the mercury contamination of their clothes. To keep the environment safe, an ISO certified Mercury Waste Amalgam Separator should be installed in the dental office to keep mercury from being dumped into the sewer system.

MERCURY DETOXIFICATION

If you have had your amalgam silver-mercury fillings for many years, you have been exposing yourself to mercury vapor during eating drinking and brushing. Since no matter what precautions are taken, a certain small amount of mercury exposure is possibly unavoidable during mercury filling removal procedure. It may be wise to protect yourself during the process of removing dental filings by taking heavy meal binding and other nutritional supplements. Some nutritional supplements can dramatically reduce and protect you from absorbing toxic materials as well as help support and optimize your organs and bodily functions. It is advisable to seek a knowledgeable health care provider in helping you come up with a strategy of heavy metal detox and supplementation. The following is a list of commonly used methods you should be familiar with.

Medical

The best way to remove mercury form your body is by chelation therapy. While IV chelation is effective, it can be expensive, time consuming and painful. A simpler approach is via suppositories. DMSA suppositories are made by a compounding pharmacy and should be taken for 3 months. Since chelation therapy removes key minerals along with heavy metals a practical approach is to administer the suppositories every other day. On days off take a double dose of a good quality multi vitamin. Repeat the urine porphoryn test after 3 months to confirm the effectiveness of chelation therapy.

Other non-medical methods of mercury detoxification are discussed below for completeness, however they may not be as effective as DMSA. Regardless of which method you chose, make sure to check your urine porphoryn levels before and after beginning any detox procedure to make sure it is effective.

Nutritional

Activated Charcoal: Activated Charcoal is one of the finest absorptive and adsorptive agents known. Orally administered, these fine black granules have an amazing ability to extract and neutralize many more times their own weight in gases, heavy metals, toxins, poisons and other chemicals. Charcoal can decrease your body's absorption of certain nutrients and also interfere with medications. Because of this, only take it immediately after amalgam removal.

Chlorella: Chlorella Pyrensioda, a single-cell green algae, that was popularized by the Japanese since the 1940's and is the top supplement in that country today. In addition to its outstanding vitamin and mineral content, it is beneficial in helping to remove heavy metals like mercury; lead and cadmium from the body. The International Academy of Oral Medicine and Toxicology (IAOMT) advises that chlorella supplementation should be started 2 weeks prior to mercury containing amalgam filling removal and continued for 2-3 months after completion.

New Nanonized Chlorella: 'Nanonized' means "very, very small." Through a revolutionary new process, broken cell wall chlorella (the most biologically available form) is micro-digested by beneficial probiotic microorganisms through a process called nanization. The nanized chlorella's highly bioavailable phytonutrients allow unmatched cellular delivery of its detoxifying factors. Thus, nanized chlorella is more capable of binding with mercury and other heavy metals released during dental amalgam removal. New research shows that "nanized chlorella" can mobilize mercury and other toxic metals rapidly from the nervous system and whole body when taken daily over a period of time (generally 2 to 3 months). The mobilized mercury is excreted through the urine, not the intestines. This is a revolutionary discovery and showcases nanized chlorella as a premier substance to mobilize mercury from the body. It is the safest, most effective natural heavy metal detoxifier (especially mercury) yet discovered. It is very effective for both children and adults, especially those with brain fog, learning, behavioral or memory challenges.

A typical, recommended daily amount is 1/2 to 1 teaspoon at breakfast and dinner, mixed in 2 to 3 oz.

water. It is best sipped slowly over several minutes (not swallowed quickly) for best absorption.

Natural Clay: Clay has been used as a medicament for healing, detoxification and nutrition since ancient times. Natural clays have a strong negative charge that binds bacteria and toxins such as heavy metal ions. These toxins are then absorbed into the clay like a sponge. The clay is not able to pass our intestinal lining due to the epithelial cells' negative surface charge. The two like charges repeal each other. The clay is eventually harmlessly eliminated through our bowels.

Support Supplements

Alpha-Lipoic Acid: ALA is powerful antioxidant that protects against damage to the body's cells and serves vital functions at the cellular level, such as energy production. ALA is an effective mercury chelator because it binds to mercury and carries it out of your body via the urine or feces.

Vitamin D: Vitamin D is critical for uptake of calcium. Taking high quality cod liver oil (which has naturally occurring vitamin D) or mushroom mycelial extracts is beneficial as they also deliver biologically active provitamin D. If supplementing, take vitamin D3 and have your vitamin D levels checked regularly. Most people are deficient in Vitamin D.

Organic Oil of Oregano: Oil of oregano is an essential oil with potent anti-inflammatory and healing properties. You can massage a drop or two into the gums to relieve inflammation or pain following dental work. For those who are sensitive to oil of oregano, organic neem oil (see below) work as well.

Organic Limonene Oil: Limonene is an essential oil extract of orange peel. Its famous anti-inflammatory and healing properties makeing it a tremendous help during dental work. It can be massaged around painful gums or teeth. Mixing a few drops of oil of oregano, limonene oil, and/or neem oil in your hand then applying it to the gums can provide deeper penetration.

CoQ-10: Much research shows the significant effects of CoQ-10 in helping to reverse periodontal disease and promote gum integrity to help save teeth. For best results, use only naturally derived, temperature-stable CoQ-10. Avoid synthetic CoQ-10, especially found as gel-caps.

Superoxide Dismutase (SOD): A new form of SOD has been naturally derived from Bifido bacteria and concentrates the rare manganese form of SOD, shown to be highly effective. Other forms of zinc based SOD have been shown to be unstable and not absorbable. The manganese form of SOD is administered sublingually for immediate absorption and reliable delivery into the blood stream. It is a premier anti inflammatory, helping to clear tissue inflammation, speed healing and clear infection. This can be a great help to speed recovery for sore or aching teeth.

Organic Neem Bark, Neem Oil, Neem Leaf Tea: Organic neem bark, oil and neem leaf tea, when free of solvents and other toxic chemicals used in processing, can deliver premier anti-inflammatory and broad-spectrum anti-infective properties that can be used long term without irritation or inflammation.

Neem is an ideal remedy when struggling to eliminate periodontal and tooth infections. A mixture of neem bark and neem oil (1/8 tsp. of bark and a few drops of oil) can be applied locally around the gums or teeth or taken internally to affect the whole body via the gastrointestinal tract.

Coral Minerals: They are rich in highly ionized, naturally occurring calcium and magnesium as well as many trace minerals. These minerals are profoundly efficient in helping to establish your pH in the alkaline zone (reflected by a 6.5 to 7.0

first-morning urine pH). To get the best results from dental work, your pH should be kept well within the alkaline range. If your pH is very acid (below 6.0), you may find dental work may be much more difficult.

A Note of Caution

Before you begin amalgam removal with an experienced and trained dentist in the IAOMT protocol, it is advisable to discuss a supplementation plan with a knowledgeable health care provider. Functional doctors, nutritionists, chiropractors and acupuncturists with nutritional degrees, doctors of Osteopathic Medicine, alternative care physicians and open-minded physicians are good resources. Most dentists that focus on safer mercury filling removal know of local health care providers who can help you with heavy metal detox and can make a recommendation to suit your needs.

TOOTH COLORED FILLINGS

Today the two most frequently used tooth colored materials to fill teeth are bonded Composite-Resin fillings and Glass Ionomer fillings. In addition to these materials, Porcelain or ceramic fillings can be used to restore teeth.

COMPOSITE-RESIN FILLINGS

Composite fillings have been in use since the 1980's. The bonding technology and resin fillings have been improving for the past 30 years. Today there are thousands of composite-resin tooth-colored materials and bonding adhesives available to dentists. Many dentists are resistant to using these materials because they are more expensive than mercury amalgam fillings, require meticulous technique and attention to detail and understanding of organic chemistry that is individual to each adhesive and composite material. Composite-resin materials are marketed to dentists based on how shiny they get and how easy they are to handle and how fast they are to place. While these properties are important, there are other more important criteria.

One major argument against composite resin fillings is that "they do not last as long as amalgam fillings". This may have been true with the early generation white fillings that wore out faster than mercury amalgam fillings; but today, materials are available that wear just like teeth. An important point to consider is that while amalgam fillings are strong, they often last at the expense of the tooth. What good is a filling if it cracks or breaks the tooth???

On the other hand, resin-composite fillings often fail because the bond between the tooth and the filling breaks and bacteria leak in, causing decay around the filling. This often occurs when the filling is not properly bonded to the tooth in the first place (technique failure). Or the resin material is too flexible relative to the tooth causing it to deform and de-bond. When the filling deforms more than the tooth during chewing, the bond between the tooth and the filling weakens and ruptures. This can lead to decay under and around the fillings and loss of the filling altogether. Being too flexible is a major shortcoming of many resin composites on the market today. Unfortunately, there are only a few composite resin materials with the same physical properties of the tooth.

Bisphenol-A in Resin Composite Fillings
And you thought all you had to worry about was the mercury in your fillings? There has been a

tremendous concern about the health effects of BPA (an estrogen mimicker) containing composite-resins in sealants and fillings. Fortunately, there are companies that manufacture BPA-free composite resin filling material

Studies have found detectable levels of BPA in the saliva of patients after they received some brands sealants or composite-resin fillings. Experts are divided as to whether this low exposure constitutes a health risk. However, a study published in the Journal of the American Dental Association in 2006, found some dental products leach BPA and could result in low-dose exposures within the range in which health effects have been seen in rodents. Although The FDA has officially cleared Bisphenol A as a public health concern, many patients remain skeptical. After all, The FDA is known to make major blunders, remember Vioxx and Z-Pack???

Fortunately, some dental companies are aware of the issue and are formulating products that do not contain or release BPA.

GLASS IONOMER FILLINGS

Glass Ionomers are another type of white filling material. While they exhibit the same thermodynamic properties as teeth, they have low bond strengths to teeth and contain fluoride, which is constantly being released into the mouth. Glass Ionomers are also weak and do not hold up well to chewing over time. Glass Ionomer fillings are traditionally used as a base under fillings and crowns, in baby teeth and elderly people with very high decay rates. If you are against fluoride containing fillings this may not be a good choice for you.

PORCELAIN FILLINGS

Porcelain or ceramic inlays are bonded into the tooth similar to a composite-resin filling. While the ceramic fillings look good, many studies have shown that bonded porcelain inlays do not last any longer than composite-resin fillings. However, the cost of porcelain filling can be 3-4 times as much as composite filling. Ceramic fillings are weak when they are thin and require a minimum thickness. Often healthy tooth structure has to be removed in order to create a deep and wide enough hole in the tooth to prevent premature fracture of the glass. In addition, there is a concern that deep porcelain filling is too rigid and do not work in harmony with the tooth. Similar to a metal filling, the rigid ceramic filling can increase the risk of tooth fracture.

Minimally Invasive Dentistry: Less is More
Teeth are not just little white rocks we chew with. They are complex, biologic structures that help us to chew, speak, smile, whistle and sometimes

defend ourselves. A wise dentist once said, "there is no dentistry better than no dentistry". What he was eluding to is that dentistry is the art of repair, and no repair is better than the original thing. A growing trend across all disciplines of dentistry is Minimally Invasive Dentistry also known as Conservation Dentistry. Minimally invasive dentistry is one of the principles of Biomimetic Dentistry.

New technologies like Advanced Magnification in the form of Prism Loupes and Surgical Microscopes combined with Air Abrasion, Tooth and Gum Lasers and specially designed micro-drills allow modern dentists to remove tooth decay and cracks in teeth with pinpoint accuracy. Dentists should make every effort to preserve the healthy parts of your teeth.

Crack Reinforcement with Fiberglass Mesh
It is common to find cracks in teeth that have mercury-silver amalgam fillings. Ideally all cracks should be removed from inside the tooth. However, if a crack extends under the gum or close to the nerve, the risks associated with crack removal are too great. Fortunately, crack repair and reinforcement is part of the Biomimetic Dental protocol. The tooth is sealed and a woven fiberglass mesh is placed over the crack. This is similar to pacing a fiberglass mesh between 2 pieces of sheetrock and spackling the mesh. Studies confirm that this approach to

repairing cracked teeth improves the tooth's strength and substantially decreases crack propagation

NON-DECAYED TOOTH "CAVITIES"

A number of destructive tooth processes result in loss of tooth structure that is not tooth decay related, yet are just as problematic for the long-term survival of your teeth. Although enamel is highly wear resistant, it is not designed to withstand the unnatural environment we have created. Once the enamel is destroyed, the softer inner dentin begins to deteriorate at a very rapid rate. Exposed dentin can be very sensitive to cold and sweets, is more prone to decay, and if allowed to progress deep enough can be the cause of nerve death. In addition, dentin destruction at the neck of the tooth, by the gum line, can cause teeth to weaken and snap off at the gum line.

Tooth Erosion

Chemical erosion of tooth structure can be a serious problem. Consumption of acidic beverages or acidic foods such as citrus fruits can often result in the chemical dissolution of enamel and dentin. Habits such as sucking on lemons, or "fruit mushing" can cause rapid destruction of tooth structure. In addition, swimmers who frequently swim in chlorinated pool water year-round can develop chemical wear of their teeth.

Systemic disease such as acid reflux, GERD and bulimia expose teeth to stomach acid, which can be extremely destructive and caused rapid tooth erosion.

Tooth Abrasion

When gums recede and expose the softer tooth root to the mouth environment, toothbrush abrasion can form concave holes in the roots. This is a slow process and can take years for the damage to occur. Most of the wear is actually caused by the toothpaste, which is a mild abrasive that is safe on enamel, but can cause wear on dentin.

Tooth Abfraction

When teeth are exposed to excessive forces, especially at an off angle as occurs with crowded and misaligned teeth stress defects can occur. The cusps of teeth are shaped like mountains, with peaks and valleys. The upper and lower teeth fit together in such a way that the peaks fit in to the valleys of opposing teeth. This creates a stable situation just like nature intended. What is common with misaligned teeth is that the tip of one cusp slams into the sides of the opposing cusp. This creates a very stressful situation in the tooth. Teeth are the most flexible at the neck of the tooth, which is at the gum line. When aberrant forces are applied, the dentin at the neck of the tooth breaks off at an angle scausing a wedge shaped defect in the root at the gum-line.

Like root abrasion these defects weaken the tooth and can cause similar symptoms of cold and sweet sensitivity, food trapping, increased decay, and risk of nerve death and the top of the tooth snapping off.

Tooth Attrition

Tooth grinding or bruxism over a prolonged period of time can cause premature tooth wear. Some patients grind so much for so long that the enamel is completely worn off their teeth exposing the softer dentin below. Once the dentist becomes exposed, it wears very rapidly creating scooped out or bowl shaped concavities in the chewing surface of the teeth. These areas are more prone to food trapping, decay and tooth sensitivity. When this occurs in the front teeth the enamel thins, becomes to long transparent and begins to chip making teeth took irregular and short.

Some dentists ignore non-decay defects, because they are not "cavities". However, as with any disease process they get worse with time. The treatment is as simple as placing a bonded filling to replace the missing dentin or enamel. Often no local anesthetic is necessary. What is more important is to address the cause of the destructive process so it does not continue to damage your natural teeth.

CROWNS

Why Do Teeth Need a Crown?

A crown (a.k.a. cap) is a protective restoration. In general, when a substantial area of your natural tooth is missing because of a large cavity or tooth breakage there is not always enough healthy remaining tooth left to hold the filling in place. Placing large fillings in such weakened teeth may cause the filling to fall out or break prematurely with added further tooth fracture, which results in a need for a crown anyway or even loss of the tooth. It is always better to treat teeth right, the first time. Repeated drilling on teeth can cause increased risk of nerve death and need for root canal therapy. It is common to see crack lines around large mercury-amalgam fillings. In fact, broken teeth with large mercury-amalgam fillings are the second most common dental emergency.

Teeth that are weakened by amalgam fillings often have vertical crack lines as well as diagonal crack lines under the cusps. When left untreated, these cracks can spread deeper into the tooth. Cracks that enter the nerve cause severe pain, nerve death and the need for Root Canal Treatment. Some cracks can spread deep into the tooth and cause the tooth to split, requiring gum surgery or extraction.

A crown serves as a protective restoration to hold the tooth together and helps prevent further breakage. This is why weak teeth with cracks or fracture lines require a crown. Think of an old fashioned wood barrel with metal rings around it. The rings serve to hold the barrel together just like a crown holds the tooth together.

Back teeth are designed to crush food and are exposed to the largest forces in the mouth. When a back tooth has had Root Canal Treatment it usually severely weakened from deep decay or large fillings. In addition, because a major source of moisture, the blood vessels, inside the tooth is removed, the tooth becomes more brittle. Think of a tree branch: a live, moist branch bends, while a dry brittle branch snaps. The standard of care is to cover the cusps of a root canal treated back chewing tooth by a protective crown in order to help prevent the tooth from splitting and breaking. It is rare to see a root canal treated tooth survive a patient's lifetime with out a protective crown.

Another reason to place a crown when large areas of the tooth are missing is to provide ideal shape to the restored tooth. It is technically difficult and sometimes impossible to create ideal tooth shape with a free-hand placed filling. Poorly shaped fillings can create areas of food entrapment or ledges, which may lead to further tooth decay or gum disease. Typically a crown requires 2-4 office visits to complete. However, an innovative technology that has been evolving over the past 28 years is the CEREC CAD/CAM system. This allows the dentist to make a strong, all-porcelain crown in just one visit. This saves people valuable time, there is no need for a temporary that may fallout and the need for multiple shots at every visit is eliminated.

Partial Crowns:

Time for a history lesson: During dentistry's infancy in the 1800's it was customary to restore teeth with partial gold crowns know as Onlays, because they covered or "overlaid" a portion of the tooth. These restorations were very tooth conservative, replacing only the damaged part of the tooth. However, because adhesive dentistry did not exist, intricate preparations and pin systems had to be used to help retain the onlay. Tooth preparations were difficult and not every dentist could master this technique.

During the 1950's technology was developed to fuse porcelain to metal much enameled pots and pans. The era of the "cosmetic crown" began. In order to help retain the new crowns, the teeth were drilled down to the shape of a thimble: a flat topped tapered-wall preparation. Thus was necessary because adhesive dentistry did not exist and mechanical retention of wedging 2 tapered objects was necessary. Think of two glasses wedged together. While more cosmetic than metal, the porcelain-fused-to metal crowns require aggressive tooth reduction. The entire protective enamel outer layer is drilled away along with some of the dentin. Studies show that crown preparation of teeth weakens them considerably and increases the likelihood of nerve death and the need for Root Canal Therapy. Crown preparations mutilate the natural tooth because they destroy otherwise healthy parts of the remaining tooth.

As adhesive dentistry matured and advances in porcelain technology improved, dentists began having the choice to once again restore teeth with partial crows or onlays. All-ceramic onlays are bonded to the tooth thereby reinforcing it. Only the decayed and weak parts of the tooth are removed, the remaining healthy tooth is preserved and the missing portion is replaced by a natural looking all-ceramic restoration that has similar wear characteristics as enamel and is kind to opposing natural teeth. Minimally invasive as well as tooth conserving porcelain onlays are the ideal way to restore teeth with missing cusps or full cusp coverage that is necessary following root canal therapy. Mutilation of healthy teeth is no longer needed to achieve an esthetically pleasing result.

New Biocompatible Ceramic

Biocompatibility is regarded as a material's quality of being compatible with the biological environment, i.e. the material's ability to interact with living tissues by causing no, or very little biological reactions. A dental material is considered to be "biocompatible" if its properties and function match the biological environment of the body and do not cause any unwanted reactions.

Based on the criteria of the protocol, IPS e.max—lithium disilicate, is considered non-cytotoxic and meets the requirements of the Agar Diffusion Test, ISO 10993-5 guidelines. A study evaluating biocompatibility of e.max concluded that lithium disilicate was greater than or equal to many commonly used dental alloys and dental restorative materials. In addition e.max is 4 times stronger than the conventional feldspathic porcelain used for crowns. E.max has very similar wear rates to enamel and does not damage opposing teeth. Monolithic crowns made form 100% e.max will not delaminate as often happens with bi-layer crowns where the porcelain is fused to a metal substructure.

Can't you just fill it, doc?

A filling requires a certain amount of tooth structure in order to stay in place. When one or more cusps are weakened or missing, and cusp replacement is required, a partial crown, onlay or crowns are better, longer lasting choices. Filling materials do not hold up long term and wear prematurely when replacing cusp. This causes teeth to drift, shift and negatively effect the bite. In addition, it is not always possible to create an ideal shape when replacing large portion of the tooth with a direct filling. Improperly shaped fillings can cause food entrapment, gum problems and increased tooth decay. Generally when more than 50% of the tooth is missing, especially a cusp, an indirect (made outside the mouth) tooth restoration is the better choice.

BIOCOMPATIBILITY TESTING

Toxicity to dental materials can occur when certain products are placed in the mouth cause that person's immune system to react and "reject" the restoration since the components are never accepted in the same manner as one's own tissues. This is probably one of the primary concerns facing dental patients today. With several thousand dental restorative materials available on the market, it is important to know how vigorously or minimally these materials will react with the body's immune system.

Serum compatibility testing provides dentists with one way to help determine which materials will react in a test tube with a patient's serum proteins, and to what extent this will happen. Proper testing can help to prevent the placement of any of a number of materials in the mouth that could prove to be an ongoing source of toxins to a patient. Reactivity to dental materials can be loosely compared to food allergies. While many people have no problems with foods such as peanuts, shellfish, or strawberries, there is a small percentage of the population who will have an allergic reaction to these foods. The reaction to dental materials that are tested for is similar to an allergy, but it can appear to be subtler. Most people do not even notice that anything is happening since they experience no immediate symptoms, but there can still be a reaction-taking place. The immune system can react to dental materials as if they were infections or just toxic substances, and it will begin to work overtime to remove the "infection" from the body, although this can obviously never occur as long as the substances remain in the mouth. Most of the time, these materials are placed with no investigation into potential problems because the dentists themselves are unaware of the hazards. While no ethical dentist would ever knowingly place a toxic material in a patient's mouth, most are simply unaware of the danger. Very few dentists are ever taught that patients can have a reaction to dental work, and those who are educated often believe that only certain types of materials are reactive, and that by avoiding them, they can avoid any such problems. The truth is that anybody can have an immune reaction to any material, and one very good way to minimize the possibility of such problems is to test the body's reactions in vitro (in a laboratory) via Serum Biocompatibility Testing.

Immune Reactivity

The human immune system is one of many methods that the body has to protect itself from harm. It works by recognizing substances that do not belong in the body and removing them. Such substances are called antigens and may include viruses, bacteria, fungi, toxins, and parasites. Immunologists describe two general types of antigens: those that are supposed to be present in the body are called "self" antigens, while those that are not supposed to be there are called "non-self" antigens. Recognition and removal of antigens is handled by about a dozen specialized cell types collectively known as white blood cells or leukocytes. It is theoretically possible for anything to create an immune response. All that needs to happen is for the immune system to recognize the substance, and the immune system can recognize any antigenic substance.

Many of the metals and components of composite materials are part of a group of chemicals called haptens. These are atoms or small molecules that do not prompt an immune response themselves, but they can combine with a carrier, a larger molecule (usually a protein) in the body, to form a substance that will trigger the immune system. If the carrier is a self-antigen then there is a possibility that the immune system will begin to recognize the carrier without the hapten. This results in an autoimmune disease, where the immune system attacks part of the body as if there were an infection. These types of immune reactions have been linked to diseases such as multiple sclerosis and lupus erythematous.

The presence of dental or other toxins in the body is easy to detect by the elevated levels of lymphocytes and other components of the immune system. One would expect to see similar elevations in a person suffering from a cold or flu. These elevations indicate that the immune system is actively fighting an infection. The difference is that with a cold or flu, the immune system can eventually rid the body of the infection. With dental toxicity, the source of the problem is permanently imbedded in the mouth and only the chemicals that are released into the body can be dealt with. This keeps the immune system on "alert" status all the time, while simultaneously using a significant portion of the body's nutrients and energy in order to maintain this level of activity.

While there are thousands of materials available for use in dental restorations, there are three major types of material: metallic, composite and ceramic.

Metals: Metallic components include both amalgam materials and casting alloys. Amalgams are used primarily as filling materials, and casting alloys find use in crowns and bridges, as bases for ceramic restorations, and in orthodontic work.

The first and perhaps the most talked about types of dental restoration materials are amalgam fillings. An amalgam is obtained by mixing mercury with other metals; this mixture can then be used to fill a cavity. The mixture is often liquid or very near to a liquid at room temperature, so it can easily form to the contours of a cavity and fill the space very effectively. Recently, an increasing number of patients are moving away from amalgam fillings for a variety of reasons: some for aesthetic reasons, others because of concerns about the mercury content or concerns over metallic components in general.

Many other dental restorations use gold or other precious metal-based casting alloys, and are most commonly used in crowns. While pure gold is much too soft to make effective dental restorations, it has many other properties that make it an ideal starting material for dental alloys. Several other metals are commonly mixed with gold in order to obtain an alloy that combines the most favorable properties of each metal. Gold and platinum are often selected because they are resistant to tarnish and corrosion and often demonstrate only very minimal immune reactivity in the biocompatibility testing. Metals like copper and palladium are used to modify the color of the alloy, while others such as silver and iridium are used to give the alloy more strength. There are even more metals that are used in dental work to alter melting points, hardness, color, and the durability of alloys. Any given alloy could have up to a dozen different component metals, so it is important to know which metals you will substantially react to before they are placed in the mouth.

Resins: Resin-Composite materials, commonly known as "white fillings," are one type of dental material that is quickly gaining popularity. These are a type of glass-plastic material, often selected for aesthetic reasons because they can be made to look just like a real tooth. Many patients prefer composite fillings because they are sensitive to the other types of fillings available. Perhaps the most common misunderstanding about composite fillings is that they are all the same. Actually there are a wide variety of component chemicals that can be used to make composites, allowing a dentist to use precisely the right material for any situation.

The plastic portion of the composite is a polymer, a large molecule that is made up of many smaller molecules called monomers. These monomers are usually a type of dimethyl acrylate that is able to form long chains, as well as links between chains to form a very stable polymer matrix, like a spider's web, that will not dissolve in water. Inside the polymer matrix is some sort of glass filler material. Quartz, borosilicate, silicon dioxide, and barium glass are among the more commonly used materials for this purpose. These fillers keep the composite from expanding or shrinking, prevent water absorption, and make the plastic stronger. Some composites also contain catalysts and accelerators to make the plastic portion set more quickly and effectively. Methacrylic acid and colloidal silica can also be added to the mixture to obtain a faster setting and stronger filling. Finally, a surface treatment is used to link the polymer and the filler together. Since there are many different options for each component, and not every component is used, there are literally thousands of possible combinations of chemicals that can make a composite material.

Ceramics: Porcelain and ceramic materials are popular as dental restoratives because they look and feel very much like real teeth. It is difficult to provide a comprehensive list of ceramic components since they vary greatly depending, not only on the materials used but also depending on the type of restoration. The basic ceramic restoration consists of the exterior restoration, which is fused to a framework. The framework is then attached to the teeth in order to hold the prosthetic in place. The exterior can be cut or milled from a prefabricated block of material, or it may be built up layer by layer to give the proper shading and appearance of a real tooth. It is then fired in order to harden the material and fuse the ceramic to the framework. The framework can be either a metal alloy (often gold based), or a sturdier form of ceramic.

The exterior ceramic is usually a type of porcelain made up of silicon dioxide, and typically containing varying amounts of zirconia or alumina to give it the proper color. Ceramic restorations can contain far more ingredients than those listed above, and the variations in composition give the wide range of properties that any given material can produce.

The framework of a ceramic restoration can be made from metal or another form of ceramic. The metal is usually an alloy of gold, platinum, palladium and silver, although many other metals are often used. A ceramic framework generally has high zirconia content and can contain any of the same components as the exterior material.

Serum Biocompatibility Testing

Serum Biocompatibility testing was developed to determine how much of an immune reaction a particular client will have to any given material. A blood sample is drawn and spun on a centrifuge in order to separate the blood cells from the blood serum. The cells are discarded and the serum, which contains all of the free-floating antibodies and other blood proteins, is collected for testing. A small sample of the serum is then mixed with the individual chemical components that may be found in dental materials. If the chemicals would cause an immune reaction in the body, then the antibodies present in the serum will bind the chemicals and form an antibody complex making the mixture look cloudy.

This is known as a protein fallout reaction. A simple but elegant machine called a light densitometer is then used to measure the opacity of each serum-chemical mixture, and the chemical is then judged according to protocols originally developed by Dr. Hal Huggins and refined over decades of testing. For the dentist's convenience the classifications "Highly Reactive," "Moderately Reactive," and "Least Reactive," are used to aid in understanding the results. Each product on the test is then rated by the highest reactivity level among its component chemicals. This assures that only the products in which all components give the lowest reaction levels are termed "Least Reactive."

If you are concerned about reactivity or allergy to dental materials, speak to your dentist about Serum Biocompatibility Testing. A well respected company is the Clifford Consulting and Research Lab which is known to perform such tests.

GUM DISEASE

Gum disease is a silent epidemic. According to several studies nearly 85% of the American population has some stage of gum disease, medically called Periodontal Disease. In addition about 50% of the population has moderate to severe periodontal disease. It is a painless disease, often unnoticed by patients until their teeth get loose or start shifting. In fact, gum disease is the number one reason we lose our teeth today in the U.S.

Losing your teeth from gum disease is just the tip of the iceberg, when it comes to your overall health. Gum disease has been implicated as a risk factor in several diseases including, obesity, heart attack and stroke, Alzheimer's and dementia, erectile dysfunction, pancreatic cancer and many more. Expecting mothers have additional risk if preeclampsia, gestational diabetes, miscarriage, pre term and low birth weight babies. The list of diseases grows yearly. Surprisingly, many people know very little about it. As the body of evidence regarding the gum disease—systemic disease connection grows and physicians become more aware of the connections, we will see more and more reports about this in the media.

The connection is inflammation. Gum disease is a chronic inflammatory disease. It adds to the overall inflammatory burden on the body. The previously mentioned diseases have one thing in common: **inflammation.** By decreasing inflammation in our bodies, we can live longer, healthier disease-free lives. Having healthy gums, free from inflammation is one step towards achieving that goal.

The standard of care is to examine every new patient for gum disease and measure the gums by performing a six-point gum measuring around every tooth on an annual basis as part of a periodic examination. Shockingly, the American Academy of Periodontology has stated that 73% of dental offices do not evaluate their patients for periodontal disease. In addition, according to the American Dental Association, 50% of the offices diagnosing gum disease do not measure the gums for severity of periodontal disease. This means that, at best, 13.5% of offices across the country are meeting the gum disease diagnostic standard of care.

Many advances have been made in the recent years to treat gum disease without surgery. Modern dentists combine all the possible treatment methods for gum disease treatment in order to help patients avoid painful gum surgery and maintain healthy gums for a lifetime.

THE FOUR STAGES OF GUM DISEASE

Healthy gums: Gums are actually attached to our teeth forming a seal around the tooth. This seal keeps the bacteria inside our mouths from entering our bodies. When gums are pink, firmly attached to your teeth, never bleed they are healthy. In addition to a visual inspection of the gums, dentists evaluate the health of your gums by measuring the space between the gum and the tooth with a round-ended ruler. Healthy gums measure between 1-3 millimeters and do not bleed or hurt during the measuring process. It is also important to evaluate your x-rays to make sure there are no tartar under the gums and no bone destruction around the roots.

Stage I gum disease: When Plaque and Tartar build up around the teeth and are not removed in a timely fashion, gum disease begins. Plaque and Tartar are full of billions of disease causing bacteria that infect the gums causing gum inflammation or Gingivitis. Inflamed gums are red, swollen and bleed easily. The good news is that Stage I Gum Disease is fully reversible with proper treatment.

Stage II Gum Disease: If not removed, the plaque and tartar deposits on the roots begin to creep deeper under the gums. This causes the gums to separate from the tooth, breaking the biologic seal. When the space between the gum and the tooth is measured, you get a reading of 4-5 millimeters.

Stage III Gum Disease: As the plaque and tartar buildup progresses further down the root, the bacteria begin to infect and destroy the jawbone supporting the tooth. When the space between the gum and the tooth is measured, you get a reading of 6-7 millimeters. Bad breath or halitosis may become noticeable at this time. Bone destruction and tartar can be seen on x-rays.

Stage IV Gum Disease: Bone destruction continues to progress in between the roots, the teeth begin to get loose or shift, bad breath is common and it may be difficult to chew. When the space between the gum and the tooth is measured, you get a reading of 8 millimeters or higher.

SUCCESS OF GUM DISEASE TREATMENT

As with any disease, gum disease treatment success depends on several factors:

Aggressiveness of the disease: Some bacteria are more aggressive than others. Some patients present with more advanced stages of disease than others. People are developing gum disease at an earlier age and the progression of disease is more advanced.

Your immune system: Nutrition, health and stress are all contributing factors in and how fast disease progresses how your body responds to treatment. For example, diabetics are at a higher risk for Gum Disease.

Genetics: Your family history plays a significant role. If your parents and grandparents had gum disease chances are that you may be at a greater risk for it as well.

Your home care: is critical for the success of the treatment. Removing Plaque daily is a fundamental requirement for success.

Your commitment to Treatment: Coming in on time and keeping your scheduled appointments is important allow dentists adequate time perform the necessary treatment. Dentists need your commitment to them so that they can help you better.

Your commitment Maintenance: Unfortunately at this time, there is no cure for gum disease. Therefore follow up care is critical. Studies show that it takes 2-3 months for the bacteria to reestablish themselves under the gums to a disease causing state. We have to constantly disrupt the biofilm that is plaque and not allow tartar to build up on your teeth. This means that missing your maintenance appointments can result in break down all over again. This can be very frustrating for you and your dentist.

OBSTICLES TO SUCCESSFUL TREATMENT OUTCOMES

The biggest obstacle to providing proper care is the patient's commitment to treatment.

The second biggest obstacle is the insurance companies. People need to be treated on individual basis depending on their specific needs. Insurance companies take the one size fits all approach, which just does not work. This may come as a surprise, but insurance companies do not care about your health, they care about their quarterly profits. You may want to watch the movie "Sicko" by Michael Moore to understand this better. Many insurance benefits are limiting. Approval for care is often done based on codes and numbers not on the patients needs. The insurance company representative does not actually see the disease going on in the patient's mouth; they do not consider your family history, health, home care, disease virulence, degree of inflammation or tartar and plaque buildup, etc. Doctors should do not be treating the insurance policy, they should be treating people! One of the biggest problems with dental insurance policies is in the area of limitation frequency of professional cleanings. The choice to receive treatment is ultimately the patient's. It is the patient's choice to follow the recommendations of the doctor or to follow what the insurance company "allows". Just do not expect the same results.

The third obstacle is the confusing medical terms and insurance codes. The glossary at the end of this book has a list of common dental terms and their definitions.

MODERN TREATMENT OF GUM DISEASE

Today many modern, minimally invasive non-surgical gum disease therapies are available. In the past decade dental lasers have become one of the fundamental innovations in gum disease treatment.

The Problem With Traditional Cut and Stitch Gum Surgery:

Traditional over 100 year old technique, which focused on periodontal pocket elimination in a resective procedure. Parts of the gums are cut away with a scalpel and are peeled off the bone so that the diseased bone can be scraped and drilled away. Then the gums are stitched back together. This mechanical removal of gum and bone procedure does little to address the real cause of the disease: the bacteria. Patients are often left with exposed tooth roots that are very sensitive, unaesthetic, and have teeth with spaces between them that act as food traps. In addition, recovery form gum surgery may include pain, swelling, bleeding, black and blue marks on the face and many stitches.

On the other hand, lasers disinfect and decontaminate the inside of the gums and address the cause of the problem: the bacteria. Laser periodontal therapy is minimally invasive, does not involve gutting away gums and bone, requires no stitches or sutures, recovery is relatively quick and comfortable with no bruising.

Early Gum Disease Laser Treatment:

When gum disease is diagnosed early and the pocked measurements range form 4-6mm, non-surgical laser periodontal therapy is effective in photo-disinfection of the infected gums around your teeth. Following a thorough deep cleaning to remove tartar, plaque and bacteria around the teeth a Diode Laser can be used to photo-disinfect or vaporize bacteria deep in the gums.

Moderate to Advanced Gum Disease Periodontal Treatment:

Currently only 2 lasers have the FDA approved Nd:Yag wavelength to treat moderate to advanced gum disease. The Periolase only uses the Nd:Yag laser, while the Powerlase or Lightwalker lasers (both made by Fotona) use both the Er:Yag and the Nd:Yag lasers in combination. The advantage of using the

Er: Yag laser in addition to the Nd:Yag laser is that the Er:Yag lase is very effective in removing all the tartar and toxins off the root surface.

For more advanced gum disease with pockets ranging 6-9mm deep Wave Optimized Periodontal Therapy (WPT) may be used. It utilizes the dual laser technique. WPT is a break through in modern minimally invasive laser periodontal treatment. By combining dentistry's two best laser wavelengths the Nd: Yag and the Er:Yag optimal results can be achieved.

The Er:Yag laser helps to remove tartar, plaque and bacterial toxins from the root surface, while the Nd:Yag laser removes diseased and infected gum tissue on the inside of the gums around the teeth, leaving the healthy outside gums intact. In addition, the Nd:Yag laser is used to form a biologic glue-clot eliminating the need for stitches. Together both lasers stimulate the bodies healing ability to help regrow healthy bone around teeth.

Oil Pulling:
Ancient Technique Makes a Comeback.

Oil Pulling is technique thousands of years old. It is a traditional remedy from ancient India that involves swishing plant oil in the mouth. It is mentioned in the Ayurvedic text Charaka Samhita where it is called Kavala Gandoosha / Kavala

Graha. A number of clinical peer reviewed studies from around the world investigated the efficacy of oil pulling and have shown a reduction in mouth bacteria and inflammation. Oil Pulling fits well into a holistic approach to dental care. Although users of oil pulling have reported both systemic and oral health benefits it is documented to improve Gum Disease (Periodontal Disease).

It is important to stress, that Oil Pulling is not a replacement for clinical removal of plaque, tartar, bacteria and bacterial toxins on the tooth above and below the gums. Oil pulling alone will not be successful and should not be used as a substitute for professional dental cleaning and gum disease treatment! It is an adjunctive synergistic therapy. By combining the best of modern dental treatments with traditional therapies that have scientific validity the result are very positive. Just as Acupuncture, Kinesiology, Chiropractic, Reflexology and Nutrition have a place in healing the body along side of modern medicine.

Although a variety of plant oils have been used, Sesame and Coconut oils are the most popular and have been used the longest. Each day take a teaspoon to a tablespoon of the oil and swish for 15-20 minutes by pushing the oil through your teeth with your tongue, chewing and moving the oil around your mouth. In the beginning your mouth will be tired, but as with any exercise you will get used to it over time. When finished, spit out the oil. It will look white and foamy. Rinse a few times with warm water.

Oil pulling is very inexpensive, has no side effects, and can help you maintain a healthy mouth as long as it is not a substitute for professional dental treatment. If you have no time to make your own Oil Pulling rinse, they are available to purchase on the Internet at **www.smithtownsmiles.com/ oil pulling**

STRESS, HORMONES AND GUM DISEASE

Recently, a strong relationship between stress and gum disease has been identified. Psychological factors such stress, depression, distress, anxiety and loneliness showed a positive relationship to periodontal disease. Scientists speculate that the hormone cortisol may be at the root of the connection between stress and gum disease. Studies have shown that elevated levels of cortisol could lead to increased destruction of the gum and jawbone around teeth due to periodontal disease. Since people under stress tend to increase their bad habits such as poor diet, poor oral hygiene and in some cases increased consumption of alcohol, nicotine or recreational drugs; they may ultimately increase their risk for a group of diseases known as Metabolic Syndrome, gum disease being among them.

Although more research in this area is needed to determine the definitive relationship some scientists believe that people who minimize stress in their lives will be at less risk for gum disease. It is suggested that by decreasing stress through healthy means such as exercise, plenty of sleep, an anti-inflammatory diet, meditation, yoga and a positive mental attitude can have a synergistic effect on the health of your mouth and gums.

WOMEN AND GUM DISEASE

Hormonal issues in women can be a significant risk factor in gum disease. Periodontal disease is often a "silent" disease; many women do not realize they have it until it reaches an advanced state. This is because hormonal fluctuations throughout a woman's life can affect many tissues, including gums. A study published in the January 1999 issue of the *Journal of Periodontology* reports that at least 23% of women ages 30 to 54 have periodontitis (an advanced state of gum disease in which there is active destruction of the gum and bone supporting the teeth). In addition, 44% of women ages 55 to 90 that still have their teeth have periodontitis.

Puberty

During puberty, an increased level of sex hormones, such as progesterone and possibly estrogen, causes increased blood circulation to the gums. This may cause an increase in the gum's sensitivity and lead to a greater reaction to any irritation, including food particles and plaque. During this time, the gums may become swollen, turn red and feel tender.

As a young woman progresses through puberty, the tendency for her gums to swell in response to irritants will lessen. However, during puberty, it is important to follow a good at-home oral hygiene regimen, including regular brushing and flossing, and regular dental care. In some cases, a dental professional may recommend periodontal therapy to help prevent damage to the tissues and bone surrounding the teeth.

Menstruation

Occasionally, some women experience menstruation gingivitis. Women with this condition may experience bleeding gums, bright red and swollen gums and sores on the inside of the cheek. Menstruation gingivitis typically occurs right before a woman's period and clears up once her period has started.

Pregnancy

Women may experience increased gingivitis or pregnancy gingivitis beginning in the second or third month of pregnancy that increases in severity throughout the eighth month. During this time, some women may notice swelling, bleeding, redness or tenderness in the gum tissue.

In some cases, gums swollen by pregnancy gingivitis can react strongly to irritants and form large lumps. These growths, called *pregnancy tumors*, are not cancerous and are generally painless. If the tumor persists, it may require surgical removal.

Studies have shown a relationship between periodontal disease and pre-term, low-birth-weight babies. Any infection, including periodontal infection, is cause for concern during pregnancy. In fact, pregnant women who have periodontal disease may be seven times more likely to have a baby that is born too early and too small. If you are planning to become pregnant, be sure to include a periodontal evaluation as part of your prenatal care.

Women who use oral contraceptives may be susceptible to the same oral health conditions that affect pregnant women. They may experience red, bleeding and swollen gums. Women who use oral contraceptives should know that taking drugs sometimes used to help treat periodontal disease, such as antibiotics, might lessen the effect of an oral contraceptive.

Gum disease can harm the developing baby. Active periodontitis has been associated with pre-eclampsia, miscarriage, preterm and low birth weight babies.

In one report, active gum infection was associated with the death of an infant. Bleeding associated with the gingivitis allowed the bacteria, normally contained to the mouth because of the body's defense system, to enter the blood and work its way to the placenta. It is suspected that the bacteria entered the immune-free amniotic fluid and was eventually ingested by the baby. A match between bacteria in the mother's mouth with the bacteria in the baby's infected lungs and stomach was made as a confirmation.

With a focus on good oral health care and preventive gum disease treatment mothers can increase their chances of giving birth to a healthy baby.

Menopause and Post-Menopause

Women who are menopausal or post-menopausal may experience changes in their mouths. They may notice discomfort in the mouth, including dry mouth, pain and burning sensations in the gum tissue and altered taste, especially salty, peppery or sour.

In addition, menopausal gingivostomatitis affects a small percentage of women. Gums that look dry or shiny bleed easily and range from abnormally pale to deep red mark this condition. Most women find that estrogen supplements help to relieve these symptoms.

Bone loss is associated with both periodontal disease and osteoporosis. Research is being done to determine whether the two are related. Women considering Hormone Replacement Therapy (HRT) to help fight osteoporosis should note that this may help protect their teeth as well as other parts of the body.

Bisphosphonate Therapy and Jaw Osteonecrosis

Bisphosphinate therapy, Fosomax Actonel and Boniva being the most popular, is used to treat osteoporosis and osteopenia and is used to help prevent bone fractures. A rare, but serious side effect of Bisphosphenate therapy is a non-healing jaw infection called Osteonecrosis. Patients who take bisphosphonate therapy for osteoporosis should be aware of this phenomenon. Surgical procedures such as tooth extractions; dental implant surgery or other bone and gum surgery should be done with caution. It is recommended that patients receiving Bisphosphonate therapy should focus on conservative dental procedures, sterile surgical technique, appropriate antibiotics and oral disinfectants prior to surgery.

GUM RECESSION

Gum recession is a common, often undiagnosed oral health problem. The simple fact is that most dentists do not view gum recession as a problem until it is too late. Common causes for gum recession are crowded teeth, tipped teeth, crooked teeth, gum disease, aggressive brushing, muscle (frenum) pull, and trauma. Gum recession is exacerbated by naturally thin bone and gums around the teeth.

A very important fact to understand that gum recession follows bone recession. That is, the gums cover the bone supporting your teeth and the only way your gums can recede is if the bone underlying the gums is destroyed. The less bone you have supporting your teeth the looser your teeth will become. This can eventually lead to tooth loss.

Common problems associated with gum recession include the following:

Tooth sensitivity: Receded gums expose the sensitive roots. Many patients complain of pain to hot or cold food and drink. Some people are also sensitive to acidic or sweet foods.

Root wear: The exposed roots are softer than enamel. Constant brushing can cause root ditching or wear. As these ditched areas get deep enough the nerve in the tooth can become compromised and die. This may result in the need for the dreaded Root Canal Treatment.

Root decay: Unlike enamel, the roots of the teeth are softer and more prone to tooth decay. In fact, in the older population root decay is the most common type of decay problem.

Esthetic issues: As the gums recede, the teeth appear to be longer. This is where the expression "long in the tooth" comes from. In some people with wide smiles the long looking teeth is a major cosmetic concern.

Loss of the protective band of gum: Around each tooth there exists a thick, fibrous band of gum called the "attached gingiva". The purpose of this gum is to protect the underlying bone and act as a seal (like a gasket) against bacteria from infecting the underlying bone. It is common to loose this protective band of gum around the lower from teeth and the middle teeth, the premolars.

Further recession: generally, unless action is taken to stop gum recession, the gums will continue to recede worsening the above mentioned problems.

Tooth Misalignment: Gum recession is often associated with crooked or misaligned teeth. When teeth are centered in the jawbone the likelihood of gum recession is less. As the teeth are pushed out of the bony housing due to rotation or misalignment, the bone around the teeth thins and the occurrence of gum recession increases. In addition, crowded, rotated and tipped teeth create increased stresses on the bone causing increased risk of gum recession. We are meant to have straight teeth. Our ancestors had straight teeth with no signs of bone thinning. Straightening your teeth to become centered in the jawbone can minimize the risk of gum recession and sometimes reverse it.

Treatment of Gum Recession

Grafting another piece of gum where recession has occurred is the only option to treat gum recession. There are several grafting options both in source of gum tissue and technique. What is best for you depends on multiple factors. The best choice for you can be determined by an experienced gum surgery specialist called a Periodontist. Gum grafting is one of the most difficult and technique sensitive dental procedures. Make sure that the dentist you choose is experienced and versed in the latest gum grafting techniques. Ask the dentist how may surgeries they have performed and what is their success rate. Some may even have before and after pictures of the teeth they treated.

Keeping your gums healthy is one of the most important things you can do to keep your teeth for a lifetime and goes a long way to keeping your overall body healthy as well.

TOOTH WHITENING

If you've already given some thought to teeth whitening, you're not alone. According to a poll conducted by the American Academy of Cosmetic Dentistry, the most common dental improvement that respondents said they'd like to have is whiter, brighter teeth. In fact, professional tooth whitening has become the most often requested procedure in many dental practices around the country.

Tooth Whitening Confusion
There seems to be an endless supply of over-the-counter and infomercial products flooding the market. As well as many dental offices offering a myriad of tooth whitening choices, so which method is right for you?

Over the Counter Products: Non-dentist supervised tooth whitening (store-bought or infomercial bought) can actually harm your teeth. Many of these products contain acid, which "frosts" your teeth making them appear whiter. This can damage the enamel on your teeth. And the actual concentration of the peroxide gel is a mystery. So you never know what you are getting.

Non-Professional One-Hour Whitening: A recent trend is to have your teeth whitened at the mall, a hair salon or on a cruise ship. Generally, a high school kid with about 1 hour of training will whiten your teeth using the one-hour light assisted technique. If you trust your teeth and gums to a quickly trained employee to apply potentially dangerous peroxide gels and hot lights to your mouth you are either brave or uninformed, so read on!

Dentist Supervised Professional Tooth Whitening: Here the choices are just as confusing. Nighttime, daytime, in office, laser whitening, light assisted whitening, 1 hour, half hour, etc. This is all very confusing, even for most dentists!

The Truth

Here is the simple fact: Real tooth whitening is achieved when the peroxide whitening gel releases oxygen into the tooth. The oxygen molecules diffuse though the enamel and break up the stain within the dentin of the tooth. The effectiveness of any tooth whitening system depends on how stained your teeth are and how <u>permeable</u> your teeth are to oxygen. Oxygen absorption into the tooth is improved by repeated exposure to the whitening gel. The oxygen release is a slow process. Tooth whitening is more dependent on how long the gel actually stays on the tooth, not how strong the gel is. The oxygen can only penetrate the tooth only so fast. It's a simple diffusion. A catalyst can make this process more effective, but lasers and lights do not. Lights are a gimmick and multiple peer-reviewed studies have repeatedly proven that!

In addition, a recent study showed that very high concentration gels that are used with light assisted whitening or laser whitening actually damage enamel, porcelain and white fillings. In fact, one hour whitening is most unpredictable whitening method today because if your teeth do not absorb oxygen well, you will have a very disappointing result that will not last. Dentists who promote laser or Light assisted whitening are either unaware of these studies and information or are consciously defrauding their patients.

At home tray tooth whitening
This method utilizes soft clear silicone trays that have been specifically made for each individual patient by taking molds of their teeth. It is important to create a seal around the gums and reservoirs for the gel. Many dentists skip these time consuming steps and results are not as good. While higher concentration daytime 1 hour and 1/2 hour gels are available, the trays are ideally worn overnight for 6-8 hours (remember contact time is very important). Usual treatment time is 2 weeks using a low-sensitivity, low-concentration peroxide gel.

This is the most effective way to use tooth-whitening trays. About 90% of patients choose this method and are very happy with the results. Some patients chose to buy more gel and continue whitening for 1-2 weeks more. Beyond 4 weeks the whitening effect plateaus and there is very little improvement beyond that. However, patients with tetracycline (antibiotic) stained teeth should continue to whiten for 4-6 months to achieve good results. This method is also very cost effective.

One-Hour In-office Power Whitening

This is the most costly method with the highest rate of side effects. The gels are typically 10 times stronger than night time whitening gels. Most dentists use a light or a laser with this method. As mentioned earlier, a light has no added benefit and is just a gimmick. Due to the unpredictable nature of this whitening method, patients may need to have additional in office treatments to achieve better results. Remember, dentists have no idea how permeable your teeth are to oxygen and there is no way to test it at this time.

Common Side Effects:

Tooth sensitivity is a common side effect. Especially in the lower front teeth. Studies have shown that the use of over the counter desensitizing toothpaste with 5% Potassium Nitrate is very effective with preventing tooth sensitivity. The higher the gel concentration, the higher the risk for tooth sensitivity. This is another reason to use low concentration nighttime whitening gels. When it occurs, tooth sensitivity is only temporary and generally does not last for more than 3 days.

Chemical burns from high concentration whitening gels may occur with sloppy technique and may result in gum burns and lip burns as well as swelling.

Caution with Mercury Fillings:

A recent study published in the prestigious *Journal of the Academy of General Dentistry* confirmed the findings of previous studies that peroxide based tooth whitening gels dramatically increase the release of mercury ion vapor from mercury-amalgam fillings. The study evaluated the lowest concentration form of tooth whitening gel containing 10% carbamide peroxide, which breaks down to 3% hydrogen peroxide. This poses a concern since frequent and prolonged exposure of amalgam to tooth whitening gels might increase the risk of mercury poisoning.

Other studies have shown that tooth whitening gels also change the physical, mechanical and structural properties of amalgam filling. This weakening of amalgam fillings can further increase mercury ion vapor release during eating, drinking and brushing.

If you are considering tooth whitening it may be advisable to replace silver-mercury amalgam fillings with resin-composite fillings to eliminate your risk for mercury exposure.

INTERNAL TOOTH BLEACHING

Sometimes root canal teeth become dark over rime. This occurs due to a break down of red blood cells from the ruptured blood vessels in the tooth. As the iron containing hemosiderin decomposes, the tooth turns a darker shade. If it is a front tooth without a crown this can become a cosmetic concern. The teeth can appear form brown to grey in color. An effective method to improve tooth color is internal tooth bleaching, a.k.a walking bleach or non-vital tooth bleaching. The filling behind the tooth is removed and a tooth whitening paste is placed inside the tooth where the top of the nerve used to be. The whitening paste is left in for several weeks as the tooth slowly returns to a normal color. Once or bi-weekly paste changes are required. This method can be used in combination with external tooth whitening to improve the over all cosmetics of the smile.

ROOT CANAL THERAPY

Common Misconceptions

Root Canal Therapy is often associated with dread and misunderstanding. In the Holistic and Alternative care community root canal therapy has been condemned for over 100 years and millions of patients may have had their teeth extracted based on what they have read from health gurus and Internet forums and websites. This chapter will examine these issues surrounding root canal therapy.

There are 2 main arguments against root canal therapy: 1. Root canal treated teeth are bastions for virulent bacteria and constantly leak bacteria and toxins into the body. 2. Root canal treated teeth are a "dead" body part and therefore should not be allowed to remain in the mouth. In order to address these concerns we need to first understand why teeth need a root canal in the first place and how it is performed today.

In the early 1900's Dr. Weston Price wrote extensively about the problems of associated with root canal therapy. His observations were very valid for his time . . . **over 100 years ago.** At that time the root canal therapy techniques, technology, science and understanding were in their infancy. Treatment outcomes were poor at best. Bacteria and pulp tissue was left in the tooth. Often large bone infections occurred causing bone necrosis, which were called "cavitations". Comparing root canal therapy of Westin Price's time to how root canal therapy can be performed at a modern dental office, using modern technology and techniques is like comparing a horse buggy to the space shuttle. Different times, different outcomes.

All root canal therapy should be performed in a clean environment using rubber dam isolation to prevent bacteria from the mouth to contaminate the inside of the tooth. This is the standard of care. In addition, the rubber dam protects the patient from accidental swallowing or inhaling of small dental instruments used during Root Canal Therapy. A Dental Microscope or high power magnification glasses should be used for improved visibility and precision. Many dentists are still using multiple x-rays to determine the length of the tooth root during treatment. Today, a mini-computer called an apex locator is used to do the same job. This minimizes x-rays during root canal treatment. Quiet electric hand pieces and the most current root canal instruments ensure a relaxed experience and less time in the dental chair.

Treatment results have become much more successful with a holistic approach and advanced disinfection protocols. The Fortona lasers Powerlase and Lightwalker are used with the PIPS protocol to thoroughly disinfect the root canal system. These Er:Yag lasers are equipped with specialized fiber optic tips. The PIPS protocol kills bacteria inside the small side branches of the root canals and within dentin tubules. Going beyond traditional rinse disinfection addresses the issue of bacteria and pulp tissue being left behind in the tooth.

The canals are sealed with a non-toxic, bio-ceramic sealer that is biocompatible to humans and deadly to bacteria as it sets. While under the clean filed, the tooth is resin sealed and a fiberglass reinforced resin composite post and core are bonded into place. This step is <u>critical</u> to ensure that no bacteria can re-contaminate the inside of the tooth. This is a departure from the traditional approach of placing a cotton ball and a leaky temporary filling after root canal therapy. Temporary fillings allow bacteria to percolate into the sealed root canal and re-infect the tooth. Studies show that once bacteria passes the temporary filling it takes 25 days for the bacterial contamination to reach the end of the root and begin causing an abscess. The fiberglass post and central filling serve to reinforce the tooth and are biomimetic, in that they have the same flexibility, compression and thermal expansion as the tooth (as opposed to metal posts and fillings). 99% of the time the entire procedure is performed in a single visit for patient convenience, comfort and significantly improved results. By completely removing the bacteria from inside the tooth, and immediately sealing the tooth form both ends the risk of re-infection and toxin build up inside the tooth is virtually eliminated.

Some people call root canal treated teeth "dead" because the nerve is removed from the inside of the tooth. This is a misnomer. Teeth are not "alive" because they have a nerve. The nerve is there to tell us that there is a problem with the tooth. This is why any stimulus to the tooth results in the sensation of PAIN. Removing the nerve, removes that sensation. However, teeth without a nerve continue to perform their physiological function in chewing, TMJ support, facial support and speech. Teeth also continue to receive moisture and sensation from the surrounding bone and ligaments even thought the main blood and nerve supply is removed. Teeth without a nerve are no more "dead" than your hair or your nails are dead (they also do not have blood or nerves). Ripping out a tooth for no other reason than it having a successful root canal treatment is highly traumatic and disruptive to the body. Healthcare providers who recommend this course of action are irresponsible, misinformed, practicing below the standard of care and are doing a huge disservice to the public.

Root canal therapy has evolved dramatically since Weston Price's time. Using 21st century technology, biocompatible dental materials, modern techniques and a holistic approach to dentistry, modern dentists can help save your teeth for a life time.

THE INS AND OUTS OF ROOTCANALTHERAPY

How Healthy Teeth Behave

The tooth is made up of two hard tissues the Dentin and the Enamel. The enamel is a rock hard outer shell of the tooth. It is a transparent-whitish tissue that is nearly 99% crystal. Enamel is the hardest tissue in our bodies and is designed to withstand the abrasive nature of chewing. Dentin makes up the inner core of the tooth as well as the roots. Dentin is 70% crystal and 30% organic and is a firm, flexible tissue similar to bone, but much denser. It is made up of millions of microscopic tunnels where tiny extensions of the nerve reside. That is why exposed dentin is "sensitive". Inside the dentin core and the roots is the Pulp. It is composed of blood vessels, which nourish the tooth, and the nerve that gives sensation to the tooth. Blood vessels and the nerve enter an exit the tooth trough a pin-sized hole at the tip of the root. The nerves in our teeth have only one sensation: PAIN!

Why Do Teeth "Die"?

The pulp lives inside the tooth, which can be thought of as a "hollow rock". Its only entry and exist is a pin-sized hole at the tip of the root. Anything that causes pulp inflammation triggers the nerve to hurt. Inflammation brings about swelling and as the tissue inside the tooth expands it has no-where to go. Given enough time or enough swelling the nerves and blood vessels inside the tooth become crushed or asphyxiated, eventually leading to nerve death. The nerve can deal with a little inflammation as when eating something very cold or hot, or a minor tap on the tooth. However, trauma, deep decay, improperly placed fillings or leaky crowns and cracks in teeth can all lead to irreversible pulp inflammation and eventual nerve death. This is a very painful process!

How Do Teeth Die?

When the pulp is inflamed and the inflammation is constant the nerve begins to die. This is often a very painful process. The pain is described as bad as the worst earache and worse that childbirth! Eventually after several days or weeks the nerve dies and the pain goes away. If you have been taking pain medicine to mask the pain and wait it out until the pain goes away, you may think everything is OK! Unfortunately, the tissue inside the tooth is silently decomposing. This is called Tissue Necrosis or Putrification. The tissue first liquefies, and then gas is released. This gas eventually begins to put pressure on the one exit: the pin-sized hole at the tip of the root. At this point pain to HOT foods or drinks is felt because the heat expands the gas, putting more pressure on the bone surrounding the tooth. The gas pressure causes the bone surrounding the root to liquefy or necrose, causing an abscess. If there is bacteria present in the tooth form a cavity, a tooth crack or poorly fitted filling or crown an infection follows. This infection can spread to the face and in rare instances to the brain. People have actually died form untreated tooth infection!

What is Root Canal Therapy?

Root Canal Therapy is the careful removal of the sick pulp from the center of the tooth and the roots, followed by disinfection and the sealing of the empty space that once housed the pulp.

Endodontists

Root canal treatment is one of the most complicated dental procedures. In fact, a Dental Specialty has been developed so that some dentists can focus their full attention and careers at performing Root Canal Treatment. These root canal specialist dentists are called Endodontists. They undergo advanced training in Root Canal Therapy as well as root canal surgery, called *apicoectomy* during a two-year post-doctorate education and training program. Root Canal Specialists spend their entire careers performing root canal treatment.

Today, with modern technology such as the dental microscope, ultrasonics, advanced disinfection procedures, lasers, improved sealing techniques and new non-toxic bioceramic cements, root canal therapy can close to 100% successful. Although some general dentists perform excellent root canal treatment, you may want to seek out a specialist who only focuses on modern root canal treatment.

LASER ROOT CANAL TREATMENT

The sad truth is that it is not uncommon for teeth that have had root canal therapy to remain infected. The persistent root canal infection is usually diagnosed months or even years after the root canal treatment was done. It is very frustrating to find out that your root canal therapy failed after having spent a large sum of money, time and possibly pain.

One of the major reasons for root canal treatment failure is that bacteria and nerve tissue not being thoroughly removed form the root canal system. Traditionally, most dentists use chemical rinses like bleach (Clorox), peroxide, chlorhexidine and iodine to disinfect and digest the tissue and bacteria inside the root. The trouble is the nerve inside the root is designed like a tree: a main trunk and many intricate branches that spread sideways. Most of the branching occurs in the last 1/3 of the root tip, but sometimes branches come from the main trunk in the mid 1/3. Dentists can only clean the main trunk with thin instruments and rely on the rinses to "take care" of the branches. Unfortunately this does not always happen even in the most experienced hands . . .

Today we finally have a dental root canal laser that can thoroughly clean all the side branches effectively and predictably: PIPS protocol with Er:Yag Fotona dental lasers and specially designed PIPS fiber optic tips. PIPS. (Photon Induced Photoacoustic Streaming) is the only proven laser root canal therapy today. Specifically, the Powerlase AT laser is the only dental laser that has been shown by several studies to completely remove all tissue and bacteria inside the tooth. *Long Island Center for Healthier Dentistry* is the only dental office on Long Island that uses PIPS during root canal therapy. Although many other dentists claim to do "Laser root canals", the lasers they use cannot achieve what the Powerlase AT PIPS has proven to do. The PIPS protocol and laser tips are a patented procedure only available to dentists who own the Fotona Er:Yag dental lasers. Just because a dentist owns a laser and sticks it into a tooth, does not mean that complete tissue and bacteria removal is achieved. In fact, no other laser has been shown to completely disinfect the entire root system.

The PIPS system is the new, revolutionary method for thoroughly cleaning the root canal system using laser energy. Harnessing this power, the PIPS laser trough a specially designed fiber optic tip creates shock waves. The laser energy pulsates through a disinfecting liquid placed inside tooth's root canal. Because the shockwaves are contained within the tooth root, the solution is able to stream through the entire canal system, thoroughly removing debris, decomposing nerve tissue and killing bacteria. As a result, the entire root canal system is left completely clean. This has been confirmed by powerful electron microscopes that can see even the smallest bacteria. The PIPS laser root canal treatment protocol even kills bacteria inside the small side branches of the root canals and within the microscopic tubules inside the tooth itself (dentin tubules). Going beyond traditional rinse disinfection addresses the issue of bacteria and pulp tissue being left behind in the tooth.

THE END OF ROOT CANALS?

Aside form trauma, most tooth nerve death arises from prolonged exposure to bacteria when tooth decay reaches the nerve. However, even if tooth decay does not reach the nerve, but is very close to it, nerve death can occur because bacteria can travel though the tiny tubules inside the dentin sand infect the nerve. Fortunately dentistry now has the understanding as well as materials necessary to avoid root canal as long as the tooth is treated in time! Many teeth may be saved from needing root canal treatment using the modern approach described next.

When a tooth is infected by bacteria tooth decay occurs. The bugs consume sugar and produce acid that slowly dissolves the tooth and allows the bacteria to invade deeper in to the tooth. There are two zones of decay: the infected layer, which is teaming with bacteria and the affected zone, which is soft and bacteria-free. A decay indicating dye, developed in Japan in 1978, can be used to stain only the infected dentin, which is then carefully removed with pinpoint accuracy with the aid of illuminated magnification and a gentle touch. In addition, new ceramic or resin burs should be used to selectively remove the infected dentin layer while leaving the affected soft dentin alone. Once all the bacteria infected dentin is removed, the tooth is thoroughly disinfected.

A new class of material: Resin Modified Calcium Silicates (RMSC) is available today to help protect the nerve and stimulate tooth healing. 10 years of research an development has resulted in Theracal-LC by Bisco, one of the leaders in dental material technology. This revolutionary material aids in the regenerative process of the tooth by stimulating dentin formation and re-mineralization of the softened affected dentin zone. In addition, this material has an alkaline pH, which is deadly to the acid loving bacteria that cause tooth decay. The material is self-sealing and adheres to the tooth forming a protective lining. If a healthy nerve is exposed during decay removal, the RMSC material provides a mechanical seal, stimulates nerve healing and secondary dentin formation. Once the deep part of the cavity, which is closest to the nerve, is treated with Theracal-LC a bonded resin-composite filling is placed. Dr. Alex Shvartsman has observed a 95% success in avoiding root canals in teeth with deep cavities and virtually no tooth sensitivity after 1 year. If you have been told you need a root canal and the nerve is still alive, you may want to get a second opinion and take advantage of today's minimally invasive, root canal eliminating technique.

DENTAL CAVITATIONS:

The term "cavitation" as it relates to the jawbones was first described in 1915 and the term was coined in the 1930's to describe the observed dead or infected hollowed out areas in the jawbone. It was presumed to have occurred due to the lack of blood supply to the bone.

In 1976 the term "cavitational osteopathosis" ("CO") was introduced. Proponents of this concept alleged that many patients had cavities within their jaws and that these cavities were not treatable with antibiotics or detectable on x-rays. During the 1980s, CO was renamed "neuralgia inducing cavitational osteonecrosis (NICO)" when pain is associated with these capitations. Some proponents of this idea locate these alleged problem areas with the unapproved ultrasound device called the Cavitat.

Some dentists who treat these NICO claim they can cure such conditions as arthritis, heart disease, and pain throughout the body by removing infected cavities within the patient's jawbones. Unfortunately, these are anecdotal and no credible scientific studies have supported this claim. The treatment advocated for CO or NICO is highly invasive and consists of drilling into the supposed "cavitations," scraping the bone and rinsing the wound with antibiotics and/or colloidal silver. The scientific evidence for both the diagnosis and treatment of CO was extremely weak. Numerous dentists performing cavitation surgery in jawbone to treat symptoms through out the body have lost their license or have been disciplined by their state boards because they were performing surgery in jawbones without any direct diagnostic evidence. Many patients of this surgery have developed infections, permanent nerve damage and disfigurement.

There does exist a true medical condition called Osteonecrosis. It is relatively new condition as is associated with a class of recent drugs called bisphosphonates (Boniva, Fosomax, etc.) which are prescribed in the treatment of osteoporosis. Patients who have tooth extractions, dental implant surgery or any other jaw bone related surgery who take bisphosphonates are at risk of developing chronically non-healing areas of bone or bone death associated with the surgical site. Dentists are well aware of this real and documented phenomenon and should take appropriate precautions.

The Weston Price Foundation (WTF) uses the words "dental foci" to describe the same hollowing out phenomenon in the jawbones. A "dental focus" is defined as an area anywhere in the mouth that is chronically irritated and/ or infected. What makes the WTF definition different is that it describes chronically infected areas in the jawbone, which is a real, well-documented and accepted phenomenon. These "dental focal infections" can include dead jaw bone areas around impacted wisdom teeth, incompletely extracted teeth, failed or re-infected root canals, infected dental implants, and teeth with a dead and necrotic nerve (from deep fillings, crowns, vertical cracks or physical trauma). What makes chronic dental focal infections so particularly difficult to diagnose is their relative lack of symptoms such as pain or swelling. According to the WPF typically dental foci "smolder" for years, manifesting only mild and intermittent symptoms of pain and swelling. This is consistent with jawbone abscess.

It is difficult to diagnose bone lesions with 2 dimensional x-rays because at least 40% of bone needs to be destroyed in order for the lesion to be visible on dental x-rays. Fortunately, a new technology is now available to dentists that allow seeing the jawbone in 3 dimensions. Unlike a CAT scan which uses huge amounts of radiation to render a 3-D image of bone, the Cone Beam Tomography (CBCT) uses low levels of radiation, about 1/4 of a complete set of x-rays, to achieve the same results. Dentists who use this technology are now able to predictably identify areas of infected bone around wisdom teeth, infected teeth, failing root canals and dental implants using this technology.

Although "cavitations" is not a recognized dental diagnosis, Dr. Shvartsman believes that what dentists of almost 100 years ago were observing, were localized bone abscesses. Now with advanced imaging technology such as the Galileos CBCT 3-D digital x-ray modern dentists are able to make the correct diagnosis and recommend proven treatment modalities. Before you have your invisible "cavitations" drilled out and scraped, risk infection, nerve damage and disfigurement you may want to have a second opinion with a proven low radiation, 3-D x-ray technology.

TOOTH EXTRACTION

The unfortunate reality is that the majority of people will have to have at least one of their permanent teeth extracted in their lifetime. There comes a point when a tooth is too badly decayed, broken down, cracked or lacking bone support due to gum disease to be saved for long term stability. As our life expectancy increases due to a healthier lifestyle or modern medicine, the chances of tooth loss increases. There are many considerations to be made if you are faced with a tooth extraction.

Tooth extraction techniques and instruments have changed little from the middle ages when your barber was your dentist and the local blacksmith made the forceps. Tooth extraction is often a brutal procedure that cracks the bone around the tooth during extraction leading to bone shrinkage of the extraction area. It took a non-dentist surgery engineer from Sweden, Gunnar Philip (the same man who designed the first laparoscopic gall bladder surgery), to redesign the tooth extraction procedure.

The Ogram technique was developed to gently remove teeth with minimal damage to the surrounding bone. Instead of ripping teeth out with brute force, the Ogram System uses newly designed instruments, and the body's own biology to free the root from the bone and gently lift the tooth out of its socket. The technique is based on a thousands year old Indian approach which uses gentle finger pressure to remove teeth. Once the biology of the process was understood, instruments were designed to facilitate this gentle tooth removal technique. Over 50% of European schools now teach this innovative modern technique and unfortunately, none in the USA.

SOCKET PRESERVATION GRAFTING

Dental implants are the standard of care in tooth replacement today. If the extracted tooth is going to be replaced by a dental implant, it would be wise to set up the site for success. It is commonly accepted as good practice to perform a socket preservation bone graft in order to help the bon heal in all 3 dimensions, thus ensuring a good future implant site.

Whether the missing tooth is replaced with a bridge, a dental implant or a denture, preserving the bone to support these restorations is critical. When a tooth is extracted the bone and the gums begin to shrink. 40% of bone is lost vertically and 60% is lost horizontally in the first 6 months and continues at a slower rate thereafter. Today tooth socket grafting is becoming the standard of care. The graft acts like a scaffold for new bone to form and the area to heal predictably. Both resorbable able and non-resorbable bone grafting is available for different situations.

The ideal time to perform a bone graft is immediately following tooth extraction. If this is not done and the bone heals poorly, performing a bone graft after the area has healed is usually more costly, involves more complicated surgery with more pain and swelling.

When missing teeth are to be replaced with dental implants, having the adequate height and width of bone is critical for successful treatment outcome. Sterilized human bone matrix has been used for decades as a predictable, safe means to graft extraction sockets. Bone stimulating proteins and collagen matrixes are now available to help speed up the bone healing process.

If a dental bridge is planned to replace the missing tooth, it is advisable to perform a non-resorbable bone graft which will prevent bone and gum shrinkage. The graft material is made form synthetic hydroxyapatite granules (Bioplant HTR). This material has over 35 years of clinical study, safety and success. In the first two years over 50% of the bone shrinks. If a bridge is placed within 2 years of extraction a space may open up under the "floating tooth" called a pontic. This will lead to annoying food impaction under the bridge, and increased risk for tooth decay and gum disease on teeth supporting the bridge.

Denture stability directly depends on good solid bone, once it is lost, the dentures become loose and unstable. In these situations placing the non-resorbing bone graft immediately after tooth extraction ensures a good quality if bone to support the denture.

Today, proteins are being developed to help stimulate bone growth within a bone graft. Research as been underway for decades and dentistry is finally seeing the fruits of these labors. Currently these proteins are very expensive, but can be used successfully in very compromised situations for predictable results. As more companies develop these proteins the price will come down, become affordable and become used more widely.

DENTAL IMPLANTS

Dental implants are now the standard of care when it comes to replacing missing teeth. Once dental implants are fused to the bone by a process called *osseointegration*, they act like anchors similar to tooth roots. Dental implants can be used to support crowns, bridges and dentures. This allows for the normal functions of speech, chewing and esthetics.

Removable partial and full dentures are the least expensive way to restore missing teeth. However many people would prefer a non-removable option. Besides the fact that they need to be removed to be cleaned, dentures may uncomfortable to wear because food constantly get sunder them causing painful mouth sores. Removable dentures transmit the chewing forces on top of the bone through the gum tissue that may hurt during chewing. Even this is something you may get used to, the danger is that these kind of forces may cause atrophy (loss) of the jawbone. Dentures are plastic and may contain acrylic, cadmium and BPA.

Dental bridges are a non-removable option to replace missing teeth. It is necessary to drill down the teeth adjacent to the missing space in order to make a bridge. Since dental implants are freestanding fixture they are tooth sparing. The cost of a 3-tooth bridge is very similar to the cost of one dental implant and crown. In fact, dental implants are more cost effective than bridges in the long term because they do not have to be replaces as often. Dental implants have a huge success rate of over 95%. That is due to the extensive amount of technology and research that go into fabricating dental implants combined with a skillful diagnosis and treatment application. Success can be improved with modern computer assisted planning and guided implant surgery. Dental insurance companies are beginning to assist with dental implant surgery and crowns.

Patients who wear partial or full dentures are great candidates for implants. You could get implants and retrofit your existing dentures over the implants. That will make a huge difference and give you the support and ability to chew most any kind of food that is a luxury that not all patients wearing dentures have!

Fortunately age is not a factor when it comes to dental implants. A patient is never too old to have dental implant treatment. With a few exceptions of severe health problems, senior patients can have implants. And is especially for our seniors, that the ability to chew and properly digest more varied and nutritious foods is very important!

While bone quantity and quality is a factor that limits the immediate implant treatment, there are bone graft and bone augmentation procedures that will allow dental implant therapy.

For those who are afraid of pain from dental impact surgery, rest assured that most patients report that it is less painful than a tooth extraction. You've probably experienced that pain when you lost your teeth. The discomfort is very easy to manage with pain medication, which is something we prescribe before and after the surgery for all of our patients. However for the truly apprehensive, in-office IV sedation is available.

THE SAFER WAY TO PLACE DENTAL IMPLANTS

Many patients do not consider dental implants because they are concerned about the surgery and risks involved to place dental implants. This concern is a real one since many vital structures such as sinuses, nerves and adjacent teeth may be damaged during free hand implant surgery.

Fortunately the days of extensive traditional surgery that can lead to major swelling and black and blue marks, pain and possible damage to nerves, adjacent teeth or sinuses are virtually a thing of the past thanks to newly available modern technology. Today, dentists can use the latest minimally invasive and safer techniques to place dental implants. Using CBCT: the 3-D low radiation digital x-ray system the jaw is scanned and a dental implant is virtually planned in the 3-D software to optimize implant size and its location in the bone relative to the future tooth. Then a surgical guide is made that will guarantee ideal implant placement based on the 3-D virtual plan. Surgical guides such as ones made by made by SICAT, a system designed by Sirona, (who makes CEREC CAD/CAM and Galileos CBCT) are within 1/5th of a millimeter accuracy of the original virtual plan. This innovative guided surgical approach reduces surgical time, large incisions, bleeding, swelling and post-surgical pain. Implants can be placed more safely, without the worry of damaging vital structures. Many patients have actually gone to work the same day!

TITANUIM DENTAL IMPLANTS

Root form dental implants were invented over 75 years ago. Over three quarters of a century these implants went through many advancements, improvements and research. Today hundreds of companies through out the world manufacture titanium dental implants. Competition had brought down the costs and has made dental implants more affordable. Most titanium dental implants are "two piece". They consist of a root shaped cylinder, which is threaded internally. A post, called an abutment, is screwed into the implant once it is fused to the bone. Finally a crown is made which is either cemented on the abutment or screwed into the implant. A common problem with early implants was screw loosening, while this can still occur today, new screw and post designs have helped to minimize this problem.

MINI DENTAL IMPLANTS

Originally designed for short-term use in supporting temporary bridges while the actual, normal size implants healed to the bone, these small diameter implants are being used today as a low-cost means to stabilize dentures and aid on Orthodontic tooth movement. These narrower dental implants are are about ½ to 1/3 the diameter of regular dental implants. Mini-implants can be used in areas of narrow bone when regular size implants are impossible, thus expanding treatment options. They have limited restorative options and are mainly used to support dentures.

ZIRCONIA DENTAL IMPLANTS

Recently, Zirconium dental have been introduced into the U.S. market. Patients with metal allergies, or those concerned about metal in their bodies now have a metal free dental implant choice.

These new innovative implants are made in an innovative manner using the Hot Isostatic Pressing Process, which removes all of the metal components and produces a strong, virtually unbreakable BioCeramic. In fact, it is three times (3X) stronger than Titanium dental implants. This amazing material is ZrO2A-TZP-BIO HIP

Another advantage of zirconium dental implants is that the post and implant are one. Most titanium dental implants require a post to be screwed into them. Titanium dental implants are hollow in the inside to accommodate the screw, making them inherently weaker and some have split or crack in this hollow weak zone. Zirconium dental implants are solid thought out and are very strong. This amazing material does not corrode, and unlike Titanium dental implants do not release metal ions into the body.

Now Zirconium dental implants come with a new surface bone-stimulating surface. This surface is laser treated to create a surface that attracts bone healing and bone forming cells from your body to allow the bone to fuse to the implant. This bioactive process is called osseointegration.

One of the major problems with traditional titanium dental implants has always been the screw loosening or screw breakage between the dental implant and the post. This is no longer an issue with the mono-block design of zirconia dental implants. Now you no longer have to worry if your crown begins to wobble form a broken or loose screw. Loose or broken screws can be a costly, time consuming and stressful matter.

Aside from the many health advantages, zirconium implants are white and do not show through thin gums. Which is common in the front area of the mouth when using black colored titanium dental implants.

Since the abutment is part of the implant, patients' do not need to spend additional money on posts, which can range form $250-$875 for prefabricated and custom implant posts, respectively. This is a significant savings if you need multiple dental implants!

The downs side of Zirconium implants is that they have only about a 10-year track record with success rated approximately 15% lower than Titanium dental implants. Which is about 80% as opposed to 95-98% for titanium implants. In addition Zirconium dental implants require a specific type of temporary to be fabricated to prevent micro-movement of the post.

Today dentists can now offer these biocompatible metal free dental implants to patients who want a metal-free option.

ALL ON FOUR: FULL ARCH RECONSTRUCTION

People who are missing all of their teeth and who hate their removable plastic dentures or people who are faced with extracting all of their teeth can benefit from this innovative full arch reconstruction approach. Developed and tested by dental implant innovating giant: Nobel Biocare. The All-On-Four protocol was developed as an affordable dental bridge option for patients who do not want to wear dentures. In addition it is possible to avoid the costly and invasive sinus lift surgery with this protocol.

Full arch dental implant restoration bridges are the most complicated dental restoration to execute. Not all dentists are trained or are familiar with its protocol. Choose a dental team that has experience with All-On-Four dental implants.

TEETH IN A DAY

When multiple implants are placed to restore a full arch of missing teeth, it is possible to attach a temporary dental bridge to the implants at the time of surgery, there by giving patients a non-removable temporary at the time of implant placement. This approach can be used with the all-on four protocol as well as when using more than four implants to restore an entire arch.

BONE GRAFTING

See chapter on Tooth Extraction for more information.

SINUS LIFT

Dental implants require a minimum amount of vertical bone height for adequate length of the synthetic root. Replacing the back upper teeth can be a challenge due to low sinuses. When the teeth are extracted and the bone shrinks, there is often an inadequate amount room to place a dental implant because the sinuses are in the way.

A specialized bone grafting technique has been developed and used for several decades. The skin under the sinus is lifted up and bone graft material is placed in the space created between the bone and the sinus skin. Over a period of 4-6 months the bone graft is converted into living bone by the body allowing dental implant placement in the upper back region of the mouth.

THE MODERN DENTAL OFFICE

Today it is an exciting time in dentistry. Advances in technology and material science are allowing dentists to provide more comfortable care with more esthetic, healthier and longer lasting dental restorations.

WHAT TO EXPECT IN A MODERN DENTAL OFFICE

Patient Education

New miniaturized intra-oral video cameras are used by modern dentists to educate patients and show them the inside of their mouth. It is said that a picture is worth a thousand words. That is why dentists are using miniature video cameras that take pictures inside the mouth and instantly transmit the images to the TV's or large monitors in the treatment rooms. No more fumbling with awkward hand mirrors! This is a helpful tool that is useful not only to educate you about your mouth, but also magnifies your teeth and aids in the diagnosis potential problems. Now patients can see their problem areas for themselves without having to "take the dentist's word for it".

Magnification Glasses

Teeth are very small, smaller than your pinky fingernail. In order to provide you with the best possible dental care dentists need to fully see what they are doing. Modern dentists wear magnification glasses called prism loupes that can magnify up to 8 times. In addition, a light can be mounted on the classes to improve visibility. If your dentist is 50 and older and is not wearing magnification glasses or even reading glasses, he/she is not seeing to the best of their ability and your dental care may suffer.

Convenience

Imagine a day when you can walk into a dental office with a broken tooth and leave with a beautiful, lifelike a all-ceramic crown, onlay or a veneer, all in just one visit. Wouldn't it be great if you no longer need to wear a plastic temporary that can fall off or break in the most inconvenient time like when you are on vacation or in a business meeting or a party? Imagine a future when you do not have to come back to the dentist two or three times to have your crown fitted. Imagine the savings in time, gas, babysitting arrangements, time off from work. Not to mention the elimination of extra injections and possible discomfort associated with additional dental visits.

That future is here and now. The technology is called Computer Assisted Design/ Computer Assisted Milling (CAD/CAM). Currently only two companies in the U.S. offer this technology: CEREC and E4D. The tooth is digitally photographed in 3 dimensions allowing the dentist to virtually design the perfect porcelain restoration for your tooth. This means no more gooey, runny rubber impression material that many patients gag on and find uncomfortable. The images are acquired in less than 30 seconds. Then using a computer controlled robotic milling machine, the crown is made right in the office. You do not have to worry that your crown is made of unknown materials in some third world country. Several materials are available including processed resin, porcelain and porcelain-resin hybrids. Unlike many traditional crown porcelains that are highly abrasive to the enamel and can prematurely wear teeth, these new materials are cosmetic and extremely strong, yet they are almost identical to tooth enamel in their abrasiveness.

Comfort

The days of gripping the dental chair and suffering through your dental visits are now in the past thanks to advances in modern dentistry. Over 50% of Americans avoid dental care entirely due to the fear of pain!

One of the most common dental phobias is being afraid of the needle. That is no surprise since the sight of a long sharp needle coming at your face is bound to send a shiver down anyone's spine. Fortunately a few modern advances have been made that make dental injections much more comfortable.

Needle-Free Injections

Dental injection without a needle is now a reality. No you are not dreaming! Needle-free dental anesthesia is a reality. The SyriJet is a device that administers dental local anesthetic with a puff of air instead of the dreaded needle. People who are afraid of a needle in their mouth really love this device. Patients experience a quick, painless "pop" from the puff of anesthetic that is delivered via pneumatic pressure into the gum. The process is over in a split second and is virtually painless.

Super Numbing Gel

To ensure a comfortable dental experience, pharmacy custom-made compounded numbing gel can be made that are more effective than commercially available numbing gels. This type of numbing gel is effective in reducing needle pain as well as reducing discomfort during professional cleanings.

Intraligamental Injections

The most difficult teeth to numb are the lower back molars. Due to the thick bone surrounding these teeth, conventional local anesthesia does not work. This is why a dental block injection is often used to numb these teeth.

This injection requires an extra long needle that is passed through the inside of the cheek, and the muscle of the face down to the bone of the inner jaw. This is one of the more difficult injections to get right and often the teeth are not adequately numb, which requires multiple injections. Sometimes patients experience an electric shock when the needle is passed near or poked into the nerve. When this happens there is a risk of nerve damage, which may result in permanent lip or tongue numbness.

Fortunately, intraligamentary injection is available that avoids the nerve block, and the risks and unpleasantness of having half of your face and tongue go numb for hours. Only the tooth that is worked on is numbed.

The dentist administers a small amount of anesthetic directly to a space between the tooth and the gums called the periodontal ligament space, rather than through the gum tissue as is usually done. Because it is so direct, we are not anesthetizing the rest of the nerves in that area, only the specific branch for that tooth.

The advantages are:

- It takes effect immediately, so there is no waiting to get numb.
- It is especially excellent for the patient who has difficulty getting numb.
- It used only a fraction of the anesthetic drug.
- It can avoid uncomfortable injections in the roof of the mouth.
- Both sides can be treated at once, avoiding additional visits.

A much more pleasant numbing experience can be achieved when the injection process starts with the needle-free SyriJet, then followed with the intraligamentary device. The numbing process is usually so smooth that the patient never feels the injection.

The Smallest Dental Needle

If a conventional injection is necessary, the dentist can chose the smallest dental needles available. Most dentists use 27 Gauge long needles to administer local anesthesia. However, 33 Gauge (the larger the gauge the smaller the needle) extra short needles are available from Germany. When combined the injection with the SyriJet needle-free injection device the result is a completely painless injection!

Computer Controlled Injection:

Besides the initial "prick" of the needle a large part of the pain associated with an injection is how rapidly the liquid is deposited under the gum. A number of devices have become available that take the injection portion of the process out of the dentists hands and is controlled by a computer. The computer slowly deposits the anesthetic. This device is useful for those dentsts that rush and do not take the care and time to slowly administer the anesthetic. It usually takes between 1-2 minutes to give a slow and painless injection.

Painless Steel

The newest advancement in needle technology is the triple bevel. The extra sharp tips glide through the tissue with very little to no discomfort. While they are more expensive, some dentists feel that the extra comfort for their patients is worth it.

VibraJet

One of the ways we make dental injections easier is by using a small, yet effective device. The VibraJet removes pain from injections based on the Gate Control Theory. The battery-operated motor easily clips onto a conventional syringe causing the needle to vibrate ever so slightly. This stimulates nerve endings and blocks the transmission of pain to the brain.

DentalVibe

An advancement over the VibraJet, the DentalVibe uses unique, microprocessor-controlled VibraPulse technology to provide the most effective way to "close" the Pain Gate to the brain and block the discomfort of dental injections. Because the brain can readily adapt to a constant stimulus, negating a closure of the pain gate, the DentalVibe is equipped with the world's first micro-processor controlled VibraPulse Technology. The micro-sonic oscillations of DentalVibe's comfort tips are pulsed in a controlled synchronized wave pattern. Along with enhanced amplitude, VibraPulse Technology sends a soothing percussive, or tapping stimulation onto the gums. This pulsed re-stimulation that maintains a closure of the gate, blocking the pain of an injection.

Articaine

A recently FDA approved local anesthetic, which has been used in Germany for over 30 years, has improved penetrating ability and faster onset. "Difficult to numb patients" are great candidates for this dental anesthetic. You will feel more relaxed knowing you will not feel a thing!

Nitrous Oxide

This safe gas can be used to reduce anxiety and stress during a dental visit. Nitrous oxide machines do not allow less than 30% oxygen, which makes it very safe since atmospheric oxygen is approximately 22 %. Although patients' are still aware, but their stress and inhibitions is reduced, similar to drinking alcohol. Once the Nitrous Oxide is turned off, patients get back to normal in about 1 minute. It is safe to drive after nitrous oxide.

Dentistry does not have to be painful or scary with today's modern technology.

Quieter Dental Experience

Electric dental drills

Traditional dental hand pieces are very loud because they use an air turbine, similar to an airplane jet engine, to power the dental drill. New electric dental hand pieces can make every patient's dental experience more pleasant. The advantages of electric hand pieces include: enhanced noise reduction, no high pitched air turbine whine, less chatter, the ability to control RPMs. They are silent quiet at low RPM.

Noise cancelling headphones

The noise of the dental drill is one of the top reasons why many patients avoid the dentist.

BOSE Noise-canceling headphones are now available that can do everything that passive ones can do—their very structure creates a barrier that blocks high-frequency sound waves. They also add an extra level of noise reduction by actively erasing lower-frequency sound waves.

These innovative headphones actually create their own sound waves that mimic the incoming noise in every respect except one: the headphone's sound waves are 180 degrees out of phase with the intruding waves. The result: the listener can focus on the sounds he wants to hear.

Laser Dentistry

A variety of dental lasers are available to treat many different dental problems.

Laser Cavity Scanner
The Diagnodent. This laser is over 90% effective in painlessly finding even the smallest cavities early.

Laser Fillings: The Er:Yag Dental Laser
This dental laser allows us to treat cavities without the use of shots and anesthetics. Over 90% of patients do not feel anything at all during treatment, and those who do say it wasn't bad enough to need a shot. You can have a filling done and go have a

meal, give a speech or meet with a client without the worry of looking and sounding funny from a numb lip and face.

Laser Early Gum Disease Treatment: Diode Laser

Photo disinfection is an effective tool to help kill bacteria in gum pockets. It has been found to be effective when used with deep cleanings, dentally called scaling and root planning.

Nd:Yag Laser for Moderate to Severe Gum Disease Treatment

Bacteria deep under your gums and around your teeth cause gum disease. Moderate and advanced gum disease is traditionally treated with surgery where the diseased gum and bone is surgically cut away. Many patients complain of tooth sensitivity and increased root cavities as well as esthetic concerns. The Nd:Yag Laser microsurgery is FDA approved as an alternative to conventional surgery. This minimally invasive technology is extremely effective at vaporizing diseased gum tissue and bacteria from around your teeth. A biologic adhesive clot is then developed with the laser to help reattach the gums back to your teeth. This is followed by Laser Bio-stimulation to speed up healing and reduce discomfort. No stitched are required.

Laser Canker Sore Treatment

Many people needlessly suffer from canker sores or aphthous ulcers. Gentle Laser energy is used to quickly heal these painful and sometimes debilitating mouth ulcers. Not only is the pain reduced immediately, but also the ulcers heal in 1 day versus the usual 10-day healing period.

Laser Cold Sore Treatment

No one likes to get a cold sore a.k.a herpes simplex I on their lip. Today cold sores can be treated successfully with lasers. In addition to topical creams and systemic medication, lasers help to reduce the duration and size of the lip infection. For best results treatment has to be initiated as soon as the lip vesicles arise and the lip feels "itchy". Once the infection has reached the crusty stage it's too late. Keep the area moist a moisturized with lip balm, coconut oil or vitamin E oil.

Laser Root Canal Therapy

Today we have a laser that can thoroughly disinfect the entire root canal system including all the side branched and dentin tubules, which typically hide bacteria. The proprietary PIPS protocol is only available with the Fotona Er:Yag Powerlase and LightWalker dental lasers. Harnessing this power of the laser with specially designed radially firing tip, the PIPS system creates shock waves within a disinfecting liquid introduced into the root canal.

Because the shockwaves are contained within the canal system, the solution is able to stream through the entire canal system, thoroughly removing debris. As a result, the entire root canal system is left completely clean, free of bacteria. You can watch this process on YouTube.com

Digital x-rays

Digital x-rays have revolutionized the dental industry. Improved diagnosis with reduced radiation is winning combination. Today two types are available.

2-D x-rays are used to diagnose cavities in between teeth and evaluate decay around fillings and crowns. The Schick 33 system is the most accurate and precise system available in dentistry today. Radiation levels can be reduced to the lowest possible setting. An estimated reduction in radiation of 98% can be achieved with Shick 33 Sensors and modern x-ray tubes as compared to traditional dental x-rays.

3-D x-rays are the latest in dental x-ray technology. They allow modern dentists to obtain a CAT Scan quality image with extremely low radiation exposure. The lower radiation machines like Galileos equal about 1 week of natural background radiation. Dentists are now able to see infections, tumors, and other difficult to diagnose problems clearly preventing major health problems for our patients. In addition, it is now possible to plan dental implants in 3-D for safer and more predictable implant surgery.

Cosmetic Dentistry

Today people are living longer and are concerned about looking and feeling younger as they age. Cosmetic Dentistry has helped many people achieve a lifetime dream of a great looking smile! It is important to note that Cosmetic Dentistry is not a recognized dental specialty and any dentist can call him/herself a cosmetic dentist. In fact, Cosmetic Dentistry is nothing more than basic modern restorative dentistry. However, there are specific attributes to look for when choosing a dentist to enhance your smile. Dentists with artistic talent, advanced training in smile design and experience in smile makeovers can excel at providing Cosmetic Dentistry to their patients. In addition, working with a talented dental ceramist that treats his craft like an art form is critical to achieving life-like, stunning cosmetic results.

Today more and more many people are realizing that how they look directly influences how others respond to them. This is true both socially and professionally. A healthy looking smile projects confidence, happiness and improves the way you look and feel about yourself. Studies have shown that a person's smile is one of the top 3 criteria people notice fist when meeting you for the first time. In fact, one study found that people with straight teeth are perceived as more intelligent than people with crowded, crooked teeth. A recent Match.com's poll also found that the smile is the #1 feature men notice most in a woman's face.

Cosmetic dentistry includes cosmetic bonding, tooth reshaping, and tooth straightening with Invisalign, porcelain laminate veneers and metal-free porcelain crowns. Tooth whitening remains the most popular cosmetic dental procedure today.

Computerized Tooth Color Matching

No more guessing your tooth color! Teeth have many different color nuances. It is important to be able to identify and match each and every tooth shade in order to get an exceptionally natural looking smile. Old fashioned methods using color tabs held against teeth require the dentists opinion and color matching skill. Fortunately, small computerized hand-held device that captures the tooth hue, value and chroma to create a color match. While these machines are extremely helpful, they are not perfect. Dentists should always corroborate the color. Women have better with color vision than men. This approach will enable you to receive the finest, most natural looking restorations that dentistry can offer.

Green Dentistry

Your dental visits can be more earth-friendly, thanks to procedures and products aimed at keeping both your mouth and our planet clean and healthy for our future. From in office procedures and products that reduce the amount of waste released into our environment to all natural toothpastes and biodegradable toothbrushes, the choices are many.

The paper-less dental practice

Computers and associated technology is allowing green-minded dentists to use digitized dental records and reduce or eliminate paper, mail, and ink cartridges, which all contribute to our planet's pollution. In fact, Congress recently passed the Health Information Technology for Economic and Clinical Health Act mandating the digitizing of all medical records by the year 2014. Dental records can be encrypted and stored safely off site for easy retrieval.

Eco-friendly x-rays

In addition to reducing X-radiation by over 90% and producing more diagnostic images digital dental X-rays are healthier for the environment. Traditional dental X-rays use led lined plastic and paper packets to store the film as well as caustic and dangerous chemicals to develop the film. Millions of gallons of these chemicals and millions of pounds of plastic and lead annually add to the pollution of our planet. Using digital x-rays may not only reduce their patient's health risks, but also help to keep our planet cleaner.

Earth-safe fillings

Traditional metal-amalgam fillings are about 55% mercury, a toxic heavy metal. In addition to heavy metal waste, there is plastic waste generated from production and disposal of plastic encased silver-mercury capsules that are used to mix the metals that produce amalgam fillings.

The flip side of the amalgam-metal filling coin is when the silver-mercury fillings are removed. Traditionally, the silver and mercury that is drilled out is simply dumped into the water system. Dental offices are the second highest cause of environmental mercury pollution. This has become such an environmental problem that several European countries, including Sweden, Finland, Denmark and Norway have banned silver-mercury fillings from use. Dentists should be using amalgam separator devices to filter the heavy metals from their water system before it reaches our environment. Every few months environmentally conscious companies carefully dispose the amalgam waste safely. Some states mandate amalgam separators in every dental office. Unfortunately these systems are expensive, compliance is low and there is little or no government oversight.

Biodegradable, recycled and earth-friendly dental supplies

As consumer demand for environment-safe products increases, companies are producing products that are made form recycled plastics and paper to biodegradable dental office supplies.

Replacing Lost Teeth

Dental implants, which are a complete tooth replacement, including the root under the gum and the tooth above the gum, are the longest lasting and most maintenance free option to replace your missing teeth. Over the course of a lifetime you will leave a smaller pollution (and financial) footprint with dental implants than dentures or bridges, which may need to be replaced every 5 to 10 years. Less maintenance and replacement over time translates into less visits to the dentist, and fewer materials and chemicals used that put a strain on our environment.

UP KEEP

MAINTENANCE

One of the single most important acts you can do to maintain your teeth healthy for a lifetime is to engage in regular professional cleaning and check-ups. Remember every disease begins as a little problem, that when caught early can be treated conservatively, with less pain, less damage and less cost.

Professional Cleanings

Most Dental Insurance Plans only cover one or two cleanings per year. One would imagine that a cleaning every 6 or 12 months is enough to maintain everyone's optimum oral health since insurance companies have your best health interests in mind, right?

Treatment, even prevention, must be based on everyone's individual needs. In order to understand this we need to look a little closer at gum disease and how to prevent it. gum disease is an infectious process caused by billions of bacteria found in dental plaque and tartar. All of us have dental plaque, which commonly forms at the gum-line. There is no way to prevent its formation on our teeth, but we can learn to remove it. Gum disease begins with red, puffy gums, which bleed easily when touched. In fact, if you brush or floss and your gums bleed you have active gum disease! As the disease progresses, the gums peel away from the teeth, bone is destroyed around the teeth and eventually teeth begin to loosen, gum abscess and bad breath become common, and teeth are ultimately lost. Remember, gum disease is the #1 reason Americans loses their teeth today and is implicated as a risk factor in many systemic diseases. A mistake many people make is avoiding professional dental cleanings allowing plaque and tartar to build up and gum disease to take hold and progress.

A professional dental cleaning is preventative procedure for *healthy gums* and is different than therapeutic gum disease treatment. Performing a preventative cleaning in the presence of moderate to advanced gum disease can cause an acute abscess and lead to tooth loss. Since gum disease severity, and progression depends on each individual's ability to remove plaque and the immune system's response to bacteria, and speed of plaque and tartar buildup. The time interval between cleanings may vary from one individual to another and within one individual at different times.

Frequency of professional dental cleanings is established with proper diagnosis. This is accomplished with thorough measurement of gum and bone levels around each tooth, taking careful note of any bleeding and abscessed areas: the sign of infected and inflamed gums, tooth mobility, bite evaluation and family history. If gum problems are discovered the first step is non-surgical treatment. How the patient responds to the treatment determines whether they are placed on a maintenance program or further therapy is necessary which may consist of antibiotic therapy or gum surgery. During each maintenance visit the dentist or dental hygienist evaluates the gums for plaque, tartar and inflammation levels. Some dentists use phase-contrast microscopes to evaluate the type of bacteria causing the disease for better diagnosis. This determines the time length between visits and need for additional gum treatment. Some require two-month intervals others can be seen every six months.

Check-ups

The standard of care is to have your teeth and mouth examined by a dentist at least every six months. A thorough dentist should only check for cavities, perform an oral cancer exam, bite exam, tooth looseness exam and update your medical history as well as discuss any concerns you have about your oral health.

X-Rays

Although many dentists take x-rays routinely every year, it is important to establish a person's risk factor in determining when to take x-rays. People with little to no tooth decay and with impeccable oral hygiene need far less frequent x-rays that someone who gets cavities all the time.

Some people refuse to take x-rays due to cost. The fact is, the cost of a crown, root canal treatment or tooth extraction and subsequent tooth replacement is far more costly than check up-x-rays and a small filling. Remember lack of pain does not equal lack of disease.

Others are worried about the effects of cumulative radiation. While this is a valid concern, dental x-rays are the lowest radiation x-rays. In addition with digital x-rays radiation exposure can be reduced by up top 98%. You get more x-rays by going outdoors! If your concern is radiation, find a modern dentist using the most recent digital dental x-rays.

Remember an ounce of prevention is worth a pound of cure!

THE FUTURE

The future of dentistry looks bright. The trend toward biomimetic, minimally invasive and tooth conserving dentistry will continue to gain ground. New developments in material science, lasers and other technology will make dentistry more comfortable, convenient and less scary. The following are some examples of technology we may see soon.

Mouth rinse to eliminate tooth decay in the future

Tooth decay is a bacterial infection of the tooth. The bacteria release acid when they consume sugar in our mouth. The acid slowly dissolves and destroys the tooth. Tooth decay rates have been increasing due to the increased processing of food and the Low-Fat Diet (High Carb) pushed by nutritionists and the government over that past decades. What people may not realize is that low-fat means high sugar. Scientists are busy trying to develop treatments to reduce tooth decay. One promising product is a mouth rinse that eliminates decay causing bacteria.

Recently, a successful clinical study involving a dozen people found that those who rinsed with the UCLA-developed mouthwash just once over a four-day testing period experienced a near-complete elimination of the *Strep. mutans*, the main decay causing bacteria. This new antimicrobial technology, can potentially wipe out tooth decay in the next several decades. More extensive clinical trials on the mouthwash are planned to start soon.

Dental ultrasound imaging technology

An innovative device is currently being developed that uses ultrasound waves for dental diagnostic purposes. The advantage of ultrasound is that it is very safe and does not emit any cancer causing ionizing radiation. Ultrasound has been safely used in the medical field for over half a century. Many people are familiar with ultrasound use for examining an unborn baby in the mother's womb. Just like the new 3-D images of the unborn baby, dental ultrasound technology will create a 3-D rendering of the tooth and its surrounding structures.

Dental ultrasound will be able to detect tooth decay in a new, more accurate way. Dentists have been using 2-D X-rays to approximate the 3-D structure of the tooth. There is a lot of "educational guessing" when reading dental x-rays. Dental ultrasound will be able to see the exact location and size of the cavity even if the cavity is between teeth (interproximal) or under and existing filling made from a metal, which is impenetrable to dental x-rays.

Currently there is no diagnostic device that has the capability of detect hairline cracks in teeth. Many patients suffer from painful tooth crack that are almost impossible to diagnose. Because ultrasound uses short wavelengths in teeth it has high resolution of fractions of a millimeter. Dental ultrasound will be very effective in detecting physical discontinuities such as fractures or cracks.

Another exciting use for dental ultrasound is its ability to penetrate various restorative materials. For the first time, dentists using ultrasound will be able to see through metal containing crowns and fillings and detect tooth decay, voids, cracks and other pathology that dental x-rays simply cannot.

Software is under development for accurately detecting Periodontal (gum) Disease. Dental ultrasound software will be able automatically measurement of the space between the gum and tooth to determine the health status of the gums. This will replace the tedious, time-consuming and often painful measuring of gums with a thin metal ruler called the perio probe. The software will automatically update the patient's electronic records easy time the dental ultrasonic scan is done.

While dental ultrasound may not completely replace dental x-rays it has diagnostic abilities that x-rays do not.

The End of Tooth Decay?

A tooth film das been developed that can mean the end of tooth decay and tooth sensitivity in the near future! Japanese scientists have invented a microscopically thin film that, when coated on teeth can prevent decay or to make them appear whiter. The "tooth patch" is a hardwearing and ultra-flexible material made from hydroxyapatite, the main mineral in tooth enamel. This innovative product can also be used to treat sensitive teeth and roots. This sheet of flexible artificial enamel can be used to protect teeth or repair damaged enamel.

The film can be made as thin as 0.004 millimeters (0.00016 inches). It becomes invisible once applied to the tooth. The hydroxyapatite sheet has a number of minute holes that allow liquid and air to escape from underneath to prevent their forming bubbles when it is applied onto a tooth. The film may be available for dental applications in as little as five years!

Bio-Engineered Natural Teeth

Dental implants could soon become a secondary choice for replacing natural teeth. The race for growing a tooth is on across the globe. We may see the fruits of this research in the next decades. In Japanese at the Tokyo University of Science scientists have successfully grown a bioengineered tooth in a mouse. In transplantation experiments a bioengineered tooth germ developed into a fully functional tooth. The tooth has sufficient hardness for mastication and exhibited nerve innervation and all the supporting structures for attachment to bone and gums. The bioengineered tooth had all the responsiveness to external stimuli as did a natural tooth. This experiment is a significant advance in regenerative therapies of artificial organ replacement.

In the U.S. at the College of Dental Medicine at Columbia University in New York, three-dimensional scaffolds infused with stem cells could yield anatomically correct teeth in as soon as nine weeks once implanted. The new technique has also shown potential to regenerate tooth-bone attachment ligaments and tooth supporting bone. This makes it possible to re-grow natural teeth that fully integrate into the surrounding tissue.

The future looks bright for replacing missing teeth with Bioengineered natural tooth replacements from stem cells or other germ cells.

Saliva Provides Early Warning Signs of Cancer

Looking inside someone's mouth may one day involve more than dental care. It could enable early diagnosis of various cancers, leading to more effective treatment outcomes and better survival rates.

Analyzing the DNA in saliva can provide clues about the molecular damage that can lead to cancer. Researchers say sampling cells in saliva could become a minimally invasive cancer screening method for large populations, and dentists might play an important role in such testing cancer patients. Although this research is in its infancy, with rapid development in DNA genetics research, we may see this test in use within a decade.

Digital Tooth Impressions.

Traditionally, dentists use a rubber-like material to take molds of teeth. Over the 30 years a new technology has been developed to take digital pictures or scans of the mouth and teeth. This means no more goop running down your throat in the future!

The first to develop this technology was Sirona for their CEREC machine. Today several companies have come out with digital surface scanning technologies. This concept is rapidly gaining ground in dentistry and some day all impressions of teeth will be done using a digital scanner. The days of gagging and worrying about chocking on the rubber materials will soon be a thing of the past in every dental office.

Stem Cells: the Future of Periodontal Disease treatment.

Several studies have already shown promising results using Bone Marrow derived stem cells in regeneration lost bone around teeth from Periodontal Disease (Gum Disease). According to a new report published in the Journal of Oral Implantology, a procedure using stem cells may provide a more thorough regeneration of periodontal tissue (cementum, bone and periodontal ligaments) around dental implants. The experimental implants received a poly-scaffold seeded with stem cells derived from bone marrow. These implants showed some level of tissue development as early as 10 days after surgery. In one month the 3 tissues required for periodontal tissue development were present. Stem Cells may play an important role in aiding bone regeneration around implants as well as bone lost due to periodontal disease

New Device Set to Nullify Dentist Drill Noise

An innovative device that cancels out the noise of the dental drill could mean the end of people's anxiety about trips to the dentist. The new invention was pioneered by researchers at Brunell University and London South Bank University. The prototype device works in a similar way to noise-cancelling headphones but is designed to specifically deal with the very high pitch of the dental drill. Patients could plug the device into their MP3 player or mobile phone, then plug their headphones into the device, allowing them to listen to their own music while completely blocking out the unpleasant sound of the drill and suction equipment. Patients can still hear the dentist and other members of the dental team, but the device filters out other unwanted sounds.

The End of Tooth Drilling?

French scientists developed a new biomaterial gel with the potential to regenerate tooth growth within cavities. This breakthrough suggests there may be new ways to treat cavities and other dental issues—without drilling and filling.

The gel is composed of a peptide called melanocyte-stimulating hormone (MSH), a compound associated with bone regeneration through studies published in the *Proceedings of the National Academy of Sciences*. Based on the theory that MSH would stimulate bone growth, the researchers combined poly-l-glutamic acid (PGL) and alpha MSH (a-MSH), resulting in PGA-a-MSH. PGA-a-MSH in gel and film forms were tested on cultures of dental pulp fibroblasts, collagen-producing cells, and other materials, and the results suggested the gel promoted regeneration and growth within these substances. The new tissue was also examined with atomic force microscopy, showing that the structure experienced increase in thickness and roughness typical of cell regeneration. When the gel was tested on the cavities of laboratory mice, the cavities were eliminated about a month later. The results confirmed that the PGA-a-MSH material increases both the viability of the cells and their ability to reproduce. INSERM researchers of the study stated that PGA-a-MSH is the first use of nanostructured and functionalized multilayered films with a-MSH for promoting endodontic regeneration.

Painless Way to Numb Teeth in the Near Future

Dental needle phobia is a common fear that many people have. This fear often results in oral health neglect and procrastination of treatment, resulting it large cavities, need for root canal treatment, infections and even tooth loss. Fortunately a new way to deliver dental anesthetics without needles is on the horizon: Aromatherapy!

A sniff of Novocain could soon replace the dental needle. Recently, scientists at Regions Hospital at Mt. Sinai, Minnesota, reported that when Lidocaine was sprayed into noses of laboratory rats, it quickly traveled to the mouth down a nerve and collected in the teeth, jaws and mouths at levels 20 times higher than in the blood or the brain. This appears to be a targeted method of numbing the mouth with low systemic effects making it an effective and safe way to deliver local dental anesthetics. The nasal spray appears to be the next generation approach beyond nasal spray in providing more rapid and targeted delivery system for oral anesthesia.

Plasma Jets Could Replace the Dental Drill

Plasmas are known as the fourth state of matter after solids, liquids and gasses. They have an increasing number of possible medical and dental applications. German scientists have showed that cold (40 C) plasma has targeted tooth decay removing properties while preserving the healthy tooth structure.

The live tissue inside the nerve is adversely affected by heat. Cold Plasma Jets, capable of obliterating tooth decay causing bacteria, could be an effective and less painful alternative to the dental drill. Research into dental applications of cold plasma jets is under way in 2 German universities and in other parts of the world. Experts estimate that clinical treatment with the Plasma Jet for dental cavities can be expected in 5-7 years.

Dr. Alex Shvartsman

Super Re-Mineralizer

Already in use in Europe, nano-hydroxyapatite toothpaste will become the best re-mineralizer available. It may replace ACP and fluoride as the king of healing cavities in the near future.

The future of dentistry is exciting for patients and dentists alike!

DENTAL GLOSSARY

In dentistry as in medicine there is terminology that is foreign even for the well-read individual. Most of the dental terms are from Latin origin, a language rarely spoken today. In order to make good health care decisions for yourself, you the patient need to understand the doctor or the dental hygienist. Dentists are not any smarter then you, they just know more about dentistry and teeth than you. If your dentist cannot speak to you in commonly understood terms, below is a glossary to decode the "dentalese" language as well as some dental jargon you may see on your bill or insurance form.

CARIES: tooth decay
CALCULUS: tartar
PALATE: roof of the mouth
INTERPROXIMAL: between the teeth
MESIAL (M): tooth surface towards the midline of the mouth
DISTAL (D): tooth surface towards the back of the mouth
BUCCAL (B): tooth surface towards the check
FACIAL (F): tooth surface towards the lips
LINGUAL (L): tooth surface towards the tongue
PALATAL (P): tooth surface towards the palate

OCCLUSAL (O): chewing surface of the tooth, top of the tooth

FISSURE: the natural groove or pit of the tooth

GINGIVA: the gums

PULP: the nerve, blood vessels inside the tooth

DENTIN: the inner core of the tooth and the root are made of this hard, yet flexible material. It is approximately 70% crystal and 30% organic

ENAMEL: the hard, rigid outer layer of the tooth that is wear resistant. It is 99% and 1% organic.

CEMENTUM: rough outer layer of the tooth into which periodontal ligaments attach.

ABFRACTION: a wedge shaped root defect caused by uneven and excessive bite forces. These non-carious lesions are the result of excessive flexing of the tooth.

PERIO PROBING: measuring the space between the gum and the tooth using a round-ended millimeter ruler.

SULCUS: The healthy space between the top of the gum and the tooth, usually measuring 1-3mm deep.

PERIODONTAL POCKET: the diseased sulcus measuring over 4mm in depth.

PERIODONTAL LIGAMENT: the millions of tiny ligaments attaching the tooth to the bone.

TOPICAL: short for "topical anesthetic": numbing gel used before injections.

INFILTRATION: injection of local anesthetic to numb the tooth.

PERIODONTAL: related to the gums.

PERIO: short for periodontal.

PROPHY: this is a name give to a professional dental cleaning. By definition it is the removal of plaque and tartar above the gum line. Most insurance companies only allow a maximum of 2 per year. A prophy is performed during your maintenance visit, it is not considered therapeutic.

PROPHYLAXIS: same as prophy.

PERIODONTAL POCKET: the diseased sulcus measuring over 4mm in depth.

GROSS DEBRIDEMENT: this is the removal of superficial tartar and plaque and debris from the teeth to facilitate healing of inflamed gums and help expose any tartar under the gums. This is a therapeutic treatment. It is always followed up by either a prophy or more advanced gum disease treatments. Unfortunately most insurance companies downgrade a Gross Debridement to a Prophy or not pay for it at all. Must be those pesky quarterly profit margins!

PERIODONTAL MAINTENANCE: essentially this is a Prophy. However patients with a history of periodontal disease are allowed by some insurance plans to have more frequent maintenance visits, up to 4 per year. They call this Periodontal Maintenance. Many insurance companies do not allow Perio Maintenance indefinitely; perhaps they want you to develop gum disease all over again.

SCALING AND ROOT PALAINING: this is the removal of plaque, tartar and bacterial waste products (toxins) deep below the gum. Specially designed ultrasonic instruments and hand instruments are used not only to remove deposits from the roots, but to smooth the roots as well. This facilitates reattachment of the gums to the roots and healing. This procedure is always done with Novocain for your comfort. Even with proper maintenance, deposits may accumulate under the gums and a deep cleaning may need to be done again in a few years.

SUB-GINGIVAL IRRIGATION: our bodies heal better without the presence bacteria. Following the physical removal of plaque, tartar and bacterial toxins from the roots. It is beneficial to irrigate below the gums with an antiseptic rinse to reduce the bacteria entering your blood. This is a safe and very effective procedure to flush out the gum pockets and rapidly reduce the bacteria numbers deep under the gums

LOCALIZED DELIVERY OF CHEMOTHERAPUTIC AGENTS: in deep pockets you may choose to have an antibiotic gel placed to further kill any remaining bacteria. Studies show that this improves healing and reattachment by as much as 62% when done in conjunction with a deep cleaning. The gel slowly dissolves over a period of 1-3 months. It has virtually no systemic effects (does not enter your body) and acts directly in the pocket itself.

PERIOSTAT: Periostat is a pill that helps to stop or slow down the progression of gum and bone break down around teeth. It is taken 2 times per day. It is a very low dose of Tetracycline. In such a low dose it does not behave like an antibiotic as it does not kill bacteria, but it does retain its gum disease fighting properties.

REFRACTORY PERIODONTITIS: relapse of gum disease. Even with proper treatment and maintenance some patients continue to have gum problems. This is very frustrating for dentists and even more frustrating for the patients. But just like any chronic disease, relapse is a reality. Sometimes disease continues despite everything we do. There are factors beyond the doctor's control such as genetics, disease virulence or a compromised immune system and patient compliance. Sometimes there are things that are difficult to control: stress, home care or nutrition.

ANTIBIOTIC PROPHYLAXIS / PREMEDICATION: antibiotics given 1 hour prior to dental treatment for at risk patients to prevent heart infection.

PERIODONTIST: gum disease specialist/surgeon

ORTHODONTIST: a dentist specializing in tooth

ENDODONTIST Root Canal Specialist, a dentist specializing in root canal therapy.

PEDODONTIST: Pediatric Dentist, a dentist specializing in treating children

ORAMAXILOFACIAL SURGEON: oral surgeon

APTHOUS ULCER: a painful white ulcer with a red border that lasts for 7-10 days.

FRENUM: the muscle fiber attachment that connects the lips and check to the gums.

FRENECTOMY/FRENULECTOMY: removal of the frenum when it causes gum recession or spaces between teeth.

INTRALIGAMENTAL: within the ligament of the tooth.

NOVOCAIN: a common name for local anesthetic. Novocain is no longer used in dentistry, but the name stuck. Common local anesthetics in use today are: Lidocaine, Marcaine, Mepivicaine, Articaine, and Prilocaine.

SEALANT: A resin coating bonded to cover deep groves in teeth that are most likely to develop cavities.

ONLAY: a metal or ceramic restoration made outside the mouth to replace one or more cusps of a tooth, sometimes called an "overlay".

INLAY: a metal or ceramic filling made outside the mouth

CROWN: also known as a "cap". A dental restoration made outside the mouth that replaces all the cusp and sidewalls of the tooth.

BRIDGE: a non-removable restoration used to replace missing tooth or teeth. Bridges are made of crowns with fake teeth fused in between them.

MARYLAND BRIDGE: a minimally invasive way to replace teeth using a face tooth suspended by flat "wings" that are glued to the back of the teeth adjacent to the space. Maryland bridges have a high failure rate and generally used as a temporary today.

ABUTMENT: a drilled down tooth or a metal implant post that is used to hold a crown that is part of a bridge.

PONTIC: the fake tooth fused between crowns on a bridge, replaces the missing tooth in a bridge.

DENTAL IMPLANT: a full tooth replacement using titanium or zirconia posts fused to the jawbone.

OSSEOINTEGRATION: the fusion of bone to a titanium or zirconium dental implant.

DENTURE: A removable appliance designed to replace some or all the teeth. It is he least expensive way to replace missing teeth. Partial dentures replace some of the teeth and use metal, resin or nylon hooks to clasp teeth for stability. Full or complete dentures replace all the teeth in the arch. Upper full dentures are retained by suction like a suction cup, while lower dentures are much less stable.

FULL MOUTH RECONSTRUCTION: The rehabilitation of a full mouth arch using a combination of crowns, bridges or dental implants.

BRUXISM: the act or habit of grinding the teeth.

PRISM LOUPES: dental magnification glasses.

GRATITUDE

It is said when the student is ready the teacher appears. I have been fortunate to come across some very special people in my life that have had a profound impact on my journey. I would like to acknowledge them here.

Robert and Tamara Shvartsman: My parents. Who gave up everything and made the difficult immigration to the USA form the Soviet Union so that their children could have the opportunity and freedom they never did.

Melissa Levin: My wife. She has been there for my greatest triumphs and biggest failures. She is my rock. Her wisdom and insight have helped me become the man I am today.

Dr. Paul Eisen: My first mentor with hands of gold. Who taught me to "become the best dentist you can be, for your self." I will cherish is teaching always.

Dr. Marc Adelberg: Whose support and friendship has helped me dream the impossible dream and make it a reality. I literally owe him my life.

Dr. Marc Cooper: Who helped me create my fantasy dental practice and become a strong leader and business owner. His wisdom and insights are priceless.

Dr. Howard Golan: Who inspired me to achieve "the next level in dentistry".

Dr. David Alleman: Who taught me Biomimetic Dentistry and changed my career forever. His personal and professional sacrifices and dedication have made a profound impact to dentistry and will improve dental care for generations to come. Hi is a true visionary and pioneer. I am fortunate to count him as a friend and mentor.

IAOMT: The organization of dentists that has taught me (and will continue to teach me) how to be a healthier dentist.

DENTISTRY WITH A PURPOSE

Whether you have been with our practice form the very inception or you are a new patient you will notice that *State of the Art Comfort Dentistry at The Long Island Center for Healthier Dentistry* is different in many unique and significant ways from the "typical" dental office. This is a story of how it came to be and a small window into the soul of my dental practice. This is form the heart.

For me, dentistry is the perfect career. It mixes my need to help people, with my interest in the sciences (especially Biology) and my natural artistic ability. I truly love being a dentist. In the late nineties when cosmetic dentistry was all the rage I spent close to a decade traveling around the country learning from the gurus of cosmetic dentistry. While I have no doubt that I helped many patients by improving their smiles, I soon discovered that there is a large number of people who have been suffering with dental fear, anxiety and full blown phobia. In fact, when people meet me for the first time and find out I am a dentist they often say, "Don't take it personally, but I HATE dentists". Well, I do take it personally, because it offends the very career that I love. While I still do a fair amount of cosmetic dentistry (in fact I believe all dentistry should be as cosmetic as possible), I decided to refocus my energy into a greater need.

In 2005 I decided to do something about people hating to go to the dentist. I stopped practicing in Glen Cove, and relocated to Smithtown, five minutes form my home so that I can be there for emergency patients quickly. Instead of just building a regular dental office, I decided that is should have a purpose. That purpose is to provide dentistry in the most comfortable manner possible and assemble a staff that genuinely cares about the people we treat. Compassion, empathy, kindness, caring and professionalism are the pillars of the office philosophy. Much thought and planning went into the decor, uniforms, equipment and technology. It was a very expensive undertaking. I zeroed out my bank account and mortgaged my home. I also took out a hefty loan. I decided to go all in, because I believed so strongly in the cause and the need of such a dental practice. I invested heavily into advanced technology to make my patients experience as comfortable as possible. Lasers, needle-free injections, digital x-rays, Nitrous Oxide in every treatment room (even for cleanings) became the norm not the exception in my every day practice. I spent 4 years at North Shore University

Hospital at Manhasset during my residency treating patients under general anesthesia. That experience allows me to confidently work with anesthesiologists to provide IV sedation or sleep dentistry in my office when the need arises.

Having a clear purpose has put every staff member into the same synchronized mind set. We all know what we are about. It's not just drilling teeth and scraping tartar. I can honestly say that I finally feel fulfilled as a doctor. I know that I am truly making a difference in peoples lives. I am grateful for my wonderful staff and the hundreds of letters form patients whose lives we have made better. Although it still makes me sad that most of the phobic patients we see are a result of my colleagues' errors, indifference or negligence. I regret to admit that, behind closed doors, phobic dental patients are often termed "pain in the ass patients" by some dentists. This attitude creates an atmosphere of annoyance and resentment. I take a different view. I realize that the stories must be heard, that more time needs to be spent listening, and that more effort has to be made to be gentle and empathetic. I will continue to buy every gadget that has the potential to improve the comfort of the dental care we provide. Some have been truly amazing, others disappointing. But it is an investment that I will continue to make in order to stay true to the purpose of *State of the Art Comfort Dentistry.*

A growing portion of my patient base is made up of people who would call themselves "holistic". If comfort is my dental practice's purpose, then holistic health would be its paradigm. I have always been into health and abide by the "do no harm" pledge. My personal holistic life style has permeated into how I practice dentistry. I have given a lot of thought into the materials I use and the type of procedures I provide. My personal belief is that nature is always better than the synthetic. Therefore, minimally invasive and tooth conserving dentistry is at the core of my dentistry. I fully appreciate that "holistic patients" want to become, and be healthy. Many have serious environmental allergies, and valid health concerns. Understandably, they find our insurance governed and Big-Pharma dominated health care system wanting. These patients are tired of the dogmatic approach of treating the symptoms with scalpels and drugs without addressing the cause of the disease and helping the body heal itself. They, like the phobic dental patients, are eschewed by many dentists who are very dismissive of their health concerns, requests and requirements. Like the phobic patients, they need to be heard and their concerns addressed. I am willing to listen, and take them seriously. In fact, I love treating my holistic patients; they are an educated consumer who does their research. In today's health care system I believe that it is important for patients to be their own health care advocates. Our office not only offers the latest in dental technology, but we also use traditional medical techniques of Herbal, Folk, Ayurvedic and Chinese medicines. In addition, I have learned so much form my holistic patients and have improved my health in the process.

"Committed to your comfort and focused on your health" has become the office mantra. I am proud of the dental practice we have created and feel very fulfilled as both a doctor and a person. Our doors and our hearts are always open to new patients and new ideas.

In good health,
Alex Shvartsman, DDS, MAGD, (AIAOMT)

ABOUT THE AUTHOR

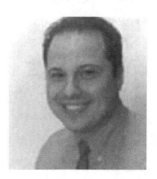

Dr. Alex Shvartsman is a dentist in Smithtown Long Island. He is a top graduate of SUNY at Stony Brook School of Dental Medicine. He also holds a BA degree in Biology from SUNY @ Stony Brook. His natural artistic talents and passion for dentistry allow him to excel as a dentist.

After completing his residency at the prestigious North Shore University Hospital at Manhasset, Dr. Shvartsman was appointed Chief Dental Resident. In addition, he has completed a two-year Fellowship in Dental Implants and Advanced Dental Prosthodontics and has taught implant dentistry at NSUH at Manhasset until his practice relocation in 2005 to Smithtown, Long Island, NY.

Dr. Shvartsman was one of the youngest Long Island dentists to have received the Fellowship Award in the Academy of General Dentistry (FAGD), by completing 500 hours of continuing education, and passing a rigorous written examination.

As a follow up, Dr. Alex Shvartsman, received the prestigious Mastership Award in the Academy of General Dentistry by completing an additional 600 hours in each required dental discipline. 400 hours were in hands-on or participation courses. He is one of a little over 1% of American dentists who have achieved this honor. Mastership in the AGD is a symbol of a dentist's continual journey toward improvement, innovation and progress. He currently serves as a peer reviewer of articles for the AGD monthly dental journal. Dr. Shvartsman's commitment to staying current in the rapidly changing field of dentistry is exemplary.

Dr. Shvartsman is the recipient of numerous additional awards, including the One of Americas Top Dentist Award, TopDocNY Award, Top Smithtown Dentist Award be the International Association of Dentists, the Suffolk County Dental Society High Level of Clinical Competence Award, and The Certificate of Merit in Recognition of Excellence and Promise in Oral Diagnosis. Dr. Shvartsman is also the winner of Long Island Press Best Dentist Award and has been featured in News Channel 12 Long Island Naturally interview.

As a nationally recognized lecturer on implant and restorative dentistry topics, Dr. Shvartsman is well respected by his peers. He mentors several young dentists on Long Island. His latest lecture on Laser Dentistry to the Westbury Dental Study Club was well received. He proudly counts other Dentists, Dental Hygienists, Dental Ceramists and their families as his patients.

He understands that the condition of your mouth affects your overall health. Dr. Shvartsman follows as Holistic Dental treatment paradigm and is proud to have never used mercury and silver-amalgam fillings and other toxic or harmful dental materials in his practice. You may have seen Dr. Shvartsman's articles on Holistic Dentistry in popular Long Island magazine s Natural Awakenings, Creations and New Living as well as his popular column "Dentally Speaking" column in various local publications. With over 15 years of dental experience you will feel confident in his gentle, caring and capable hands.

As the current president of the Long Island CEREC Forum, Dr. Shvartsman is responsible for helping to organize the study club that is devoted to advancing the knowledge and expertise of CEREC

CAD/CAM users on Long Island, including Queens, Brooklyn, Nassau, and Suffolk.

Dr. Shvartsman has been focused on Cosmetic Dentistry since being accepted in the cosmetic dentistry elective in dental school. He as been a mercury-free dentist since graduating from his residency program. In addition, Dr. Shvartsman is one of only approximately 200 dentists in the United Stated who graduated from the Alleman-Deliperi Center for Biomimetic Dentistry. He is committed to dental principles and techniques in restoring teeth as healthfully, conservatively and as naturally looking as possible. Dr. Shvartsman is a co-founder of the Academy of Biomimetic Dentistry.

Dr. Shvartsman has successfully passed the written and oral exam towards his Accreditation in the IAOMT and will be receiving his Accreditation Award at the next IAOMT meeting in Sept 2014. He also serves on the Education Committee in the IAOMT.

Dr. Shvartsman is proud to be a member of: Academy of General Dentistry (AGD), Academy of Biomimetic Dentistry (ABD), and the International Academy of Oral Medicine and Toxicology (IAOMT).

He lives St. James with his wife Melissa, their son Logan and their Burman cats Cuddles and Snuggles. Besides dentistry and his family, Dr. Shvartsman's interests include Nutrition, Reading, Hiking, Stand Up Paddle boarding, Archery and Clamming.

FURTHER READING
AND REFERENCES

Support for information in this book is contained in the following books, dental literature and peer reviewed professional journals.

BOOKS

The Paleo Solution by Robb Wolf
The Primal Blueprint by Mark Sisson
The Paleo Diet by Lauren Cordain
The Paleo Answer by Lauren Cordain
The Primal Connection by Mark Sisson
Super Immunity by Dr. Joel Furman
The Poison in Your Teeth by Tom McGuire
Mercury Detoxification by Tom McGuire
Healthy Teeth-Healthy Body by Tom McGuire

PROFESSIONAL JOURNALS

Caries diagnosis using light fluorescence devices: VistaProof and DIAGNOdent. Betrisey E, Rizcalla N, Krejci I, Ardu S. Odontology. 2013 Mar 7.

A comparative evaluation of DIAGNOdent and caries detector dye in detection of residual caries in prepared cavities. Akbari M, Ahrari F, Jafari M. J Contemp Dent Pract. 2012 Jul 1;13(4):515-20.

Caries clinical trial methods for the assessment of oral care products in the 21st century. Ellwood RP, Goma J, Pretty IA. Adv Dent Res. 2012 Sep;24(2):32-5.

Three-dimensional imaging in periodontal diagnosis—Utilization of cone beam computed tomography. Mohan R, Singh A, Gundappa M. J Indian Soc Periodontol. 2011 Jan;15(1):11-7.

Intraoral digital radiography: elements of effective imaging. Cederberg R. Compend Contin Educ Dent. 2012 Oct;33(9):656-8

Quality assurance in digital dental radiography—justification and dose reduction in dental and maxillofacial radiology. Hellstern F, Geibel MA. Int J Comput Dent. 2012;15(1):35-44.

Is it true that the radiation dose to which patients are exposed has decreased with modern radiographic films? Alcaraz M, Parra C, Martínez Beneyto Y, Velasco E, Canteras M. Dentomaxillofac Radiol. 2009 Feb;38(2):92-7.

US mortality rates for oral cavity and pharyngeal cancer by educational attainment. Chen AY, DeSantis C, Jemal A. Arch Otolaryngol Head Neck Surg. 2011 Nov;137(11):1094-9.

Association between age and high-risk human papilloma virus in Mexican oral cancer patients. González-Ramírez I, Irigoyen-Camacho M, Ramírez-Amador V, Lizano-Soberón M, Carrillo-García A, García-Carrancá A, Sánchez-Pérez Y, Méndez-Martínez R, Granados-García M, Ruíz-Godoy L, García-Cuellar C. Oral Dis. 2013 Jan 11.

Immunotherapy in new pre-clinical models of HPV-associated oral cancers. Paolini F, Massa S, Manni I, Franconi R, Venuti A. Hum Vaccin Immunother. 2013 Jan 7;9(3).

The role of human papillomavirus in oral squamous cell carcinoma. Gogilashvili K, Shonia N, Burkadze G. Georgian Med News. 2012 Dec;(213):32-6.

Papillary squamous cell carcinoma of the mandibular gingiva. Terada T. Int J Clin Exp Pathol. 2012;5(7):707-9. Epub 2012 Sep 5.

Effects of Tongue Coating and Oral Health on Halitosis Among Dental Students. Evirgen S,

Kamburoğlu K.
Oral Health Prev Dent. 2013 Mar 15.

The effect of zinc acetate and magnolia bark extract added to chewing gum on volatile sulfur-containing compounds in the oral cavity.
Porciani PF, Grandini S.
J Clin Dent. 2012;23(3):76-9.

The prevalence of periodontitis in the US: forget what you were told. Papapanou PN. J Dent Res. 2012 Oct;91(10):907-8.

New developments in tools for periodontal diagnosis. Agrawal P, Sanikop S, Patil S. Int Dent J. 2012 Apr;62(2):57-64.

Association between atherosclerosis and periodontitis López NJ, Chamorro A, Llancaqueo M. Rev Med Chil. 2011 Jun;139(6):717-24

Association between chronic periodontitis and vasculogenic erectile dysfunction. Sharma A, Pradeep AR, Raju P A. J Periodontol. 2011 Dec;82(12):1665-9.

Obesity and oral health—is there an association? Prpić J, Kuis D, Pezelj-Ribarić S. Coll Antropol. 2012 Sep;36(3):755-9.

Will periodontal treatment prevent heart disease and stroke? Merchant AT. J Evid Based Dent Pract. 2012 Dec;12(4):212-5.

Association among oral health, apical periodontitis, CD14 polymorphisms, and coronary heart disease in middle-aged adults. Pasqualini D, Bergandi L, Palumbo L, Borraccino A, Dambra V, Alovisi M, Migliaretti G, Ferraro G, Ghigo D, Bergerone S, Scotti N, Aimetti M, Berutti E. J Endod. 2012 Dec;38(12):1570-7.

Non-surgical periodontal therapy reduces coronary heart disease risk markers: a randomized controlled trial. Bokhari SA, Khan AA, Butt AK, Azhar M, Hanif M, Izhar M, Tatakis DN.
J Clin Periodontol. 2012 Nov;39(11):1065-74

Caries detection using light-based diagnostic tools. Rechmann P, Rechmann BM, Featherstone JD. Compend Contin Educ Dent. 2012 Sep;33(8):582-4, 586, 588-93

Light propagation through teeth containing simulated caries lesions. Vaarkamp J, ten Bosch JJ, Verdonschot EH. Phys Med Biol. 1995 Aug;40(8):1375-87.

The application of vizilite in oral cancer.
Sambandham T, Masthan KM, Kumar MS, Jha A. J
Clin Diagn Res. 2013 Jan;7(1):185-6.

Oral brush biopsy analysis by MALDI-ToF Mass
Spectrometry for early cancer diagnosis. Maurer K,
Eschrich K, Schellenberger W, Bertolini J, Rupf S,
Remmerbach TW.
Oral Oncol. 2013 Feb;49(2):152-6

Mucosal brush biopsy of the oral cavity to detect
local, peanut-specific immunoglobulin E. Reisacher
WR, Cohen JC. Int Forum Allergy Rhinol.
2013 Mar 20

Characterization of volatile sulfur compound
production by Solobacterium moorei.
Tanabe S, Grenier D. Arch Oral Biol. 2012
Dec;57(12):1639-43.

Dietary carbohydrates and dental-systemic diseases.
Hujoel P. J Dent Res. 2009 Jun;88(6):490-502.

Dietary habits and the state of the human oral
cavity in the prehistoric age. Taehan Chikkwa Uisa
Hyophoe Chi. 1990 Jun;28(6):555-8.

Long-term effect of maternal xylitol exposure on
their children's caries prevalence. Thorild I, Lindau

B, Twetman S. Eur Arch Paediatr Dent. 2012 Dec;13(6):305-7.

Effect of xylitol on dental caries and salivary Streptococcus mutans levels among a group of mother-child pairs. Hanno AG, Alamoudi NM, Almushayt AS, Masoud MI, Sabbagh HJ, Farsi NM. J Clin Pediatr Dent. 2011 Fall;36(1):25-30.

Caries prevention with xylitol lozenges in children related to maternal anxiety. A demonstration project. Olak J, Saag M, Vahlberg T, Söderling E, Karjalainen S.
Eur Arch Paediatr Dent. 2012 Apr;13(2):64-9.

Nonfluoride caries-preventive agents: new guidelines. Pickett FA. J Contemp Dent Pract. 2011 Nov 1;12(6):469-74.

Xylitol and caries prevention. Hanson J, Campbell L. J Mass Dent Soc. 2011 Summer;60(2):18-21.

Position of the Academy of Nutrition and Dietetics: the impact of fluoride on health. Palmer CA, Gilbert JA; Academy of Nutrition and Dietetics. J Acad Nutr Diet. 2012 Sep;112(9):1443-53.

Systemic fluoride.
Sampaio FC, Levy SM. Monogr Oral Sci. 2011;22:133-45.

Mechanisms of action of fluoride for caries control. Buzalaf MA, Pessan JP, Honório HM, ten Cate JM. Monogr Oral Sci. 2011;22:97-114.

Is systemic fluoride supplementation for dental caries prevention in children still justifiable? Oganessian E, Lencová E, Broukal Z. Prague Med Rep. 2007;108(4):306-14

The effective use of fluorides in public health. Jones S, Burt BA, Petersen PE, Lennon MA. Bull World Health Organ. 2005 Sep;83(9):670-6.

Are you drinking your teeth away? How soda and sports drinks dissolve enamel. Buyer DM. J Indiana Dent Assoc. 2009 Summer;88(2):11-3.

The erosive potential of soft drinks on enamel surface substrate: an in vitro scanning electron microscopy investigation. Owens BM, Kitchens M. J Contemp Dent Pract. 2007 Nov 1;8(7):11-20.

Effect of carbonated beverages, coffee, sports and high energy drinks, and bottled water on the in vitro erosion characteristics of dental enamel. Kitchens M, Owens BM. J Clin Pediatr Dent. 2007 Spring;31(3):153-9.

The prevalence of periodontitis in the US: forget what you were told. Papapanou PN. J Dent Res. 2012 Oct;91(10):907-8. Epub 2012 Aug 30

New developments in tools for periodontal diagnosis. Agrawal P, Sanikop S, Patil S. Int Dent J. 2012 Apr;62(2):57-64

Clinical indicators of periodontal disease in patients with coronary heart disease: a 10 years longitudinal study. Machuca G, Segura-Egea JJ, Jiménez-Beato G, Lacalle JR, Bullón P.
Med Oral Patol Oral Cir Bucal. 2012 Jul 1;17(4):e569-74.

Oral health and type 2 diabetes. Leite RS, Marlow NM, Fernandes JK. Am J Med Sci. 2013 Apr;345(4):271-3.

Level of information about the relationship between diabetes mellitus and periodontitis—results from a nationwide diabetes information program. Weinspach K, Staufenbiel I, Memenga-Nicksch S, Ernst S, Geurtsen W, Günay H.
Eur J Med Res. 2013 Mar 11;18:6.

Effect of contingent electrical stimulation on jaw muscle activity during sleep: A pilot study with a randomized controlled trial design. Jadidi F,

Castrillon EE, Nielsen P, Baad-Hansen L, Svensson P.
Acta Odontol Scand. 2012 Nov 13

Effect of conditioning electrical stimuli on temporalis electromyographic activity during sleep. Jadidi F, Castrillon E, Svensson P. J Oral Rehabil. 2008 Mar;35(3):171-83.

Human papillomavirus 16-associated cervical intraepithelial neoplasia in humans excludes CD8 T cells from dysplastic epithelium. Trimble CL, Clark RA, Thoburn C, Hanson NC, Tassello J, Frosina D, Kos F, Teague J, Jiang Y, Barat NC, Jungbluth AA. J Immunol. 2010 Dec 1;185(11):7107-14

The activity against Ehrlich's ascites tumors of doxorubicin contained in self assembled, cell receptor targeted nanoparticle with simultaneous oral delivery of the green tea polyphenol epigallocatechin-3-gallate.
Ray L, Kumar P, Gupta KC. Biomaterials. 2013 Apr;34(12):3064-76

Dental care throughout pregnancy: what a dentist must know. Achtari MD, Georgakopoulou EA, Afentoulide N. Oral Health Dent Manag. 2012 Dec;11(4):169-76.

Dental care during pregnancy Luc E, Coulibaly N, Demoersman J, Boutigny H, Soueidan A. Schweiz Monatsschr Zahnmed. 2012;122(11):1047-63

Emotional contagion of dental fear to children: the fathers' mediating role in parental transfer of fear. Lara A, Crego A, Romero-Maroto M. Int J Paediatr Dent. 2012 Sep;22(5):324-30.

Nutritional status and systemic inflammatory activity of colorectal patients on symbiotic supplementation. de Oliveira AL, Aarestrup FM. Arq Bras Cir Dig. 2012 Jul-Sep;25(3):147-53

A structural equation modelling approach to explore the role of B vitamins and immune markers in lung cancer risk. Baltar VT, Xun WW, Johansson M, Ferrari P, Chuang SC, Relton C, Ueland PM, Midttun O, Slimani N, Jenab M, Clavel-Chapelon F, Boutron-Ruault MC, Fagherazzi G, Kaaks R, Rohrmann S, Boeing H, Weikert C, Bueno-de-Mesquita B, Boshuizen H, van Gils CH, Onland-Moret NC, Agudo A, Barricarte A, Navarro C, Rodríguez L, Castaño JM, Larrañaga N, Khaw KT, Wareham N, Allen NE, Crowe F, Gallo V, Norat T, Krogh V, Masala G, Panico S, Sacerdote C, Tumino R, Trichopoulou A, Lagiou P, Trichopoulos D, Rasmuson T, Hallmans G, Roswall N, Tjønneland A, Riboli E, Brennan P, Vineis P. Eur J Epidemiol. 2013 Mar 27.

Immune function is related to adult carotenoid and bile pigment levels, but not dietary carotenoid access during development, in female mallard ducks. Butler MW, McGraw KJ. J Exp Biol. 2013 Mar 26

Remineralization of dental enamel by saliva in vitro. Koulourides T, Feagin F, Pigman W. Ann N Y Acad Sci. 1965 Sep 30;131(2):751-7.

Analysis of Dentin/Enamel Remineralization by a CPP-ACP Paste: AFM and SEM Study. Poggio C, Lombardini M, Vigorelli P, Ceci M. Scanning. 2013 Feb 20

Novel amelogenin-releasing hydrogel for remineralization of enamel artificial caries. Fan Y, Wen ZT, Liao S, Lallier T, Hagan JL, Twomley JT, Zhang JF, Sun Z, Xu X.
J Bioact Compat Polym. 2012 Nov;27(6):585-603.

An Innovative Approach to Treat Incisors Hypomineralization (MIH): A Combined Use of Casein Phosphopeptide-Amorphous Calcium Phosphate and Hydrogen Peroxide-A Case Report. Mastroberardino S, Campus G, Strohmenger L, Villa A, Cagetti MG. Case Rep Dent. 2012;2012:379593.

Casein phosphopeptide-amorphous calcium phosphate: a remineralizing agent of enamel. Gurunathan D, Somasundaram S, Kumar S. Aust Dent J. 2012 Dec;57(4):404-8.

Penetration coefficients of commercially available and experimental composites intended to infiltrate enamel carious lesions. Paris S, Meyer-Lueckel H, Cölfen H, Kielbassa AM. Dent Mater. 2007 Jun;23(6):742-8.

Does DIAGNOdent provide a reliable caries-removal endpoint? Neves AA, Coutinho E, De Munck J, Lambrechts P, Van Meerbeek B. J Dent. 2011 May;39(5):351-60.

Current concepts and techniques for caries excavation and adhesion to residual dentin. de Almeida Neves A, Coutinho E, Cardoso MV, Lambrechts P, Van Meerbeek B. J Adhes Dent. 2011 Feb;13(1):7-22.

A systematic approach to deep caries removal end points: the peripheral seal concept in adhesive dentistry. Alleman DS, Magne P.

Addressing the caries dilemma: detection and intervention with a disclosing agent. Styner D, Kuyinu E, Turner G. Gen Dent. 1996 Sep-Oct;44(5):446-9.

Fabrication and characterization of biomimetic ceramic/polymer composite materials for dental restoration. Petrini M, Ferrante M, Su B. Dent Mater. 2013 Apr;29(4):375-81.

Nanodentistry: combining nanostructured materials and stem cells for dental tissue regeneration. Mitsiadis TA, Woloszyk A, Jiménez-Rojo L. Nanomedicine (Lond). 2012 Nov;7(11):1743-53.

It should not be about aesthetics but tooth-conserving dentistry. Magne P. Br Dent J. 2012 Aug;213(4):189-91

Fatigue resistance and crack propensity of large MOD composite resin restorations: direct versus CAD/CAM inlays. Batalha-Silva S, de Andrada MA, Maia HP, Magne P. Dent Mater. 2013 Mar;29(3):324-31.

Computer-aided-design/computer-assisted— manufactured adhesive restoration of molars with a compromised cusp: effect of fiber-reinforced immediate dentin sealing and cusp overlap on fatigue strength. Magne P, Boff LL, Oderich E, Cardoso AC. J Esthet Restor Dent. 2012 Apr;24(2):135-46

Novel-design ultra-thin CAD/CAM composite resin and ceramic occlusal veneers for the treatment of

severe dental erosion. Schlichting LH, Maia HP, Baratieri LN, Magne P.
J Prosthet Dent. 2011 Apr;105(4):217-26.

Bio-emulation: biomimetically emulating nature utilizing a histo-anatomic approach; structural analysis. Bazos P, Magne P.
Eur J Esthet Dent. 2011 Spring;6(1):8-19.

Influence of overlay restorative materials and load cusps on the fatigue resistance of endodontically treated molars. Magne P, Knezevic A.
Quintessence Int. 2009 Oct;40(9):729-37.

Composite resin reinforced with pre-tensioned glass fibers. Influence of prestressing on flexural properties. Schlichting LH, de Andrada MA, Vieira LC, de Oliveira Barra GM, Magne P.
Dent Mater. 2010 Feb;26(2):118-25.

Premolar cuspal flexure as a function of restorative material and occlusal contact location. Magne P, Oganesyan T. Quintessence Int. 2009 May;40(5):363-70.

Optical integration of incisoproximal restorations using the natural layering concept. Magne P, So WS. Quintessence Int. 2008 Sep;39(8):633-43.

Direct dentin bonding technique sensitivity when using air/suction drying steps. Magne P, Mahallati R, Bazos P, So WS. J Esthet Restor Dent. 2008;20(2):130-8

Immediate dentin sealing supports delayed restoration placement. Magne P, So WS, Cascione D. J Prosthet Dent. 2007 Sep;98(3):166-74.

Immediate dentin sealing of onlay preparations: thickness of pre-cured Dentin Bonding Agent and effect of surface cleaning.
Stavridakis MM, Krejci I, Magne P.
Oper Dent. 2005 Nov-Dec;30(6):747-57.

Immediate dentin sealing improves bond strength of indirect restorations. Magne P, Kim TH, Cascione D, Donovan TE. J Prosthet Dent. 2005 Dec;94(6):511-9.

Composite resins and bonded porcelain: the postamalgam era? Magne P. J Calif Dent Assoc. 2006 Feb;34(2):135-47.

Immediate dentin sealing: a fundamental procedure for indirect bonded restorations. Magne P. J Esthet Restor Dent. 2005;17(3):144-54; discussion 155.

Analysis of factors associated with cracked teeth. Seo DG, Yi YA, Shin SJ, Park JW. J Endod. 2012 Mar;38(3):288-92

Dental composite fillings and bisphenol A among children: a survey in South Korea. Chung SY, Kwon H, Choi YH, Karmaus W, Merchant AT, Song KB, Sakong J, Ha M, Hong YC, Kang D. Int Dent J. 2012 Apr;62(2):65-9.

Time-related bisphenol-A content and estrogenic activity in saliva samples collected in relation to placement of fissure sealants. Arenholt-Bindslev D, Breinholt V, Preiss A, Schmalz G. Clin Oral Investig. 1999 Sep;3(3):120-5.

Proximal direct composite restorations and chairside CAD/CAM inlays: marginal adaptation of a two-step self-etch adhesive with and without selective enamel conditioning. Bortolotto T, Onisor I, Krejci I. Clin Oral Investig. 2007 Mar;11(1):35-43.

Single crowns versus conventional fillings for the restoration of root filled teeth. Fedorowicz Z, Carter B, de Souza RF, Chaves CA, Nasser M, Sequeira-Byron P. Cochrane Database Syst Rev.

Virtual prototyping of adhesively restored, endodontically treated molars. Magne P. J Prosthet Dent. 2010 Jun;103(6):343-51.

[Histomorphologic reactions of the teeth and parodontium to preparation for metalloceramic crowns]. Rakhlenko AG.
Biull Eksp Biol Med. 1981 Aug;92(8):101-3.

Histological pulp changes after preparation for a jacket crown. Action of an inpregnating solution on the pulp of teeth ground for jacket crowns. Blahova Z, Neumann M.
Quintessence Int Dent Dig. 1973 May;4(5):23-7.

Histological changes of the pulp after preparation for a jacket crown. The effect of an impregnating solution on the pulp of teeth prepared for jacket crowns. Blahova Z, Neumann M.
Quintessenz. 1973 Mar;24(3):41-5.

Fracture resistance of endodontically treated maxillary premolars restored with CAD/CAM ceramic inlays. Hannig C, Westphal C, Becker K, Attin T.
J Prosthet Dent. 2005 Oct;94(4):342-9.

Clinical performance of all-ceramic inlay and onlay restorations in posterior teeth. Beier US, Kapferer I, Burtscher D, Giesinger JM, Dumfahrt H.
Int J Prosthodont. 2012 Jul-Aug;25(4):395-402.

A systematic review of ceramic inlays in posterior teeth: an update. Pol CW, Kalk W. Int J Prosthodont. 2011 Nov-Dec;24(6):566-75.

Direct or indirect restorative dentistry—a mere choice about cost in relation to longevity? Waning A. Dent Update. 2011 Jan-Feb;38(1):5-10.

The longevity of direct and indirect posterior restorations is uncertain and may be affected by a number of dentist-, patient-, and material-related factors. Goldstein GR.
J Evid Based Dent Pract. 2010 Mar;10(1):30-1.

Ceramic inlays: a case presentation and lessons learned from the literature. Boushell LW, Ritter AV. J Esthet Restor Dent. 2009;21(2):77-87.

Clinical evaluation of posterior composite restorations: the 10-year report. Gaengler P, Hoyer I, Montag R. J Adhes Dent. 2001 Summer;3(2):185-94

Fluoride concentration, mutans streptococci and lactobacilli in plaque from old glass ionomer fillings. Forss H, Näse L, Seppä L. Caries Res. 1995;29(1):50-3.

Comparative clinical study of the effectiveness of different dental bleaching methods—two year follow-up. Mondelli RF, Azevedo JF, Francisconi AC, Almeida CM, Ishikiriama SK. J Appl Oral Sci. 2012 Jul-Aug;20(4):435-43.

The effect of light on tooth whitening: a split-mouth design. Henry R, Bauchmoyer S, Moore W, Rashid R. Int J Dent Hyg. 2012 Jul 12.

Clinical trial assessing light enhancement of in-office tooth whitening. Kugel G, Ferreira S, Sharma S, Barker ML, Gerlach RW. J Esthet Restor Dent. 2009;21(5):336-47.

Effect of light activation on tooth sensitivity after in-office bleaching. Kossatz S, Dalanhol AP, Cunha T, Loguercio A, Reis A. Oper Dent. 2011 May-Jun;36(3):251-7

Effect of light irradiation on tooth whitening: enamel microhardness and color change. Gomes MN, Francci C, Medeiros IS, De Godoy Froes Salgado NR, Riehl H, Marasca JM, Muench A. J Esthet Restor Dent. 2009;21(6):387-94.

Effect of in-office bleaching on color and surface roughness of composite restoratives. Hafez R, Ahmed D, Yousry M, El-Badrawy W, El-Mowafy O. Eur J Dent. 2010 Apr;4(2):118-27.

Effects of combined use of light irradiation and 35% hydrogen peroxide for dental bleaching on human enamel mineral content. Berger SB, Cavalli V, Martin AA, Soares LE, Arruda MA, Brancalion ML, Giannini M.
Photomed Laser Surg. 2010 Aug;28(4):533-8.

A randomized clinical trial comparing at-home and in-office tooth whitening techniques: A nine-month follow-up. Giachetti L, Bertini F, Bambi C, Nieri M, Scaminaci Russo D.
J Am Dent Assoc. 2010 Nov;141(11):1357-64.

Dental whitening—revisiting the myths. Perdigão J. Northwest Dent. 2010 Nov-Dec;89(6):19-21, 23-6

ER:YAG laser for 3-dimensional debridement of canal systems: use of photon-induced photoacoustic streaming. DiVito E, Lloyd A. Dent Today. 2012 Nov;31(11):122, 124-7.

Evaluation of dentin root canal permeability after instrumentation and Er:YAG laser application.
Pecora JD, Brugnera-Júnior A, Cussioli AL, Zanin F, Silva R.
Lasers Surg Med. 2000;26(3):277-81.

The antimicrobial efficacy of the erbium, chromium:yttrium-scandium-gallium-garnet laser with radial emitting tips on root canal dentin walls infected with Enterococcus faecalis. Gordon W, Atabakhsh VA, Meza F, Doms A, Nissan R, Rizoiu I, Stevens RH. J Am Dent Assoc. 2007 Jul;138(7):992-1002.

Comparison of dentin root canal permeability and morphology after irradiation with Nd:YAG, Er:YAG, and diode lasers. Esteves-Oliveira M, de Guglielmi CA, Ramalho KM, Arana-Chavez VE, de Eduardo CP.
Lasers Med Sci. 2010 Sep;25(5):755-60.

Evaluation of Nd:YAG and Er:YAG irradiation, antibacterial photodynamic therapy and sodium hypochlorite treatment on Enterococcus faecalis biofilms.
Meire MA, Coenye T, Nelis HJ, De Moor RJ. Int Endod J. 2012 May;45(5):482-91.

Two-dimensional changes and surface characteristics from an erbium laser used for root canal preparation. Roper MJ, White JM, Goodis HE, Gekelman D. Lasers Surg Med. 2010 Jul;42(5):379-83.

Irrigation in endodontics. Haapasalo M, Shen Y, Qian W, Gao Y. Dent Clin North Am. 2010 Apr;54(2):291-312

Alveolar Resorption after tooth Extraction with two different Extraction Methods A Comparison Study. Javier M. Herrera, Joachim E. Zöller, Helmut Steveling, Helmut Steveling, Dr. med. dent. Quintessence. Volume 52, pages 863-868 September

The Ögram System—a Contribution to Minimize Trauma for Tooth Extraction. Prof. Frank Peter Strietzel, Gunnar Philipp Zusammenfassung Synopsis, page 693

Current status of low intensity pulsed ultrasound for dental purposes. Rego EB, Takata T, Tanne K, Tanaka E. Open Dent J. 2012;6:220-5.

Adult Human Gingival Epithelial Cells as a Source for Whole-tooth Bioengineering. Angelova Volponi A, Kawasaki M, Sharpe PT. J Dent Res. 2013 Apr;92(4):329-34.

Perfused culture of gingival fibroblasts in a degradable/polar/hydrophobic/ionic polyurethane (D-PHI) scaffold leads to enhanced proliferation and metabolic activity.
Cheung JW, Rose EE, Paul Santerre
J. Acta Biomater. 2013 Feb 13. doi:pii: S1742-7061(13)00067-6

Regeneration of dental pulp/dentine complex with a three-dimensional and scaffold-free stem-cell sheet-derived pellet. NaS, ZhangH, HuangF, WangW, DingY, LiD, JinY. J Tissue Eng Regen Med. 2013 Jan 31

Functional Tooth Restoration by Allogeneic Mesenchy—mal Stem Cell-based Bio-root Regeneration in Swine. Wei F, Song T, Ding G, Xu J, Liu Y, Liu D, Fan Z, Zhang C, Shi S, Wang S. Stem Cells Dev. 2013 Jan 30.

Anti-caries DNA vaccine-induced secretory immunoglobulin A antibodies inhibit formation of Streptococcus mutans biofilms in vitro. Huang L, Xu QA, Liu C, Fan MW, Li YH.
Acta Pharmacol Sin. 2013 Feb;34(2):239-46

A New Approach to the All-on-Four Treatment Concept Using Narrow Platform NobelActive Implants. Babbush CA, Kanawati A, Brokloff J. J Oral Implantol. 2013 Feb 11.

Use of cone beam computed tomography and a laser intraoral scanner in virtual dental implant surgery: part 1. Lee CY, Ganz SD, Wong N, Suzuki JB. Implant Dent. 2012 Aug;21(4):265-71.

Notes concerning an overdenture on 2 implants as the standard for treating an edentulous mandible. Wismeijer D, ten BC, Schulten EA. Ned Tijdschr Tandheelkd. 2011 Dec;118(12):633-9.

In selected sites, short, rough-surfaced dental implants are as successful as long dental implants: a critical summary of Pommer B, Frantal S, Willer J, Posch M, Watzek G, Tepper G. Impact of dental implant length on early failure rates: a meta-analysis of observational studies. J Clin Periodontol 2011;38(9):856-863. Balevi B. J Am Dent Assoc. 2013 Feb;144(2):195-6.

In selected sites, short, rough-surfaced dental implants are as successful as long dental implants: a critical summary of Pommer B, Frantal S, Willer J, Posch M, Watzek G, Tepper G. Impact of dental implant length on early failure rates: a meta-analysis of observational studies. J Clin

Dr. Alex Shvartsman

Periodontol 2011;38(9):856-863. Balevi B. J Am
Dent Assoc. 2013 Feb;144(2):195-6.

Accuracy of ceramic restorations made with
two CAD/CAM systems. Hamza TA, Ezzat HA,
El-Hossary MM, Katamish HA, Shokry TE,
Rosenstiel SF.
J Prosthet Dent. 2013 Feb;

Full mouth rehabilitation for a patient with
dentinogenesis imperfecta: A clinical report.
Bencharit S, Byrd WC, Mack CR, Border MB, Wright
JT.
J Oral Implantol. 2013 Jan 4.

Three-dimensional fit of lithium disilicate partial
crowns in vitro. Schaefer O, Kuepper H, Sigusch
BW, Thompson GA, Hefti AF, Guentsch A.
J Dent. 2013 Mar;41(3):271-7.

Fracture load of monolithic CAD/CAM lithium
disilicate ceramic crowns and veneered zirconia
crowns as a posterior implant restoration. Kim JH,
Lee SJ, Park JS, Ryu JJ.
Implant Dent. 2013 Feb;22(1):66-70.

Mechanical, biological and clinical aspects of
zirconia implants. Van Dooren E, Calamita M,
Calgaro M, Coachman C, Ferencz JL, Pinho C, Silva
NR. Eur J Esthet Dent. 2012 Winter;7(4):396-417.

Effect of oil pulling on halitosis and microorganisms causing halitosis: a randomized controlled pilot trial. Asokan S, Kumar RS, Emmadi P, Raghuraman R, Sivakumar N.

J Indian Soc Pedod Prev Dent. 2011 Apr-Jun;29(2):90-4.

Mechanism of oil-pulling therapy—in vitro study. Asokan S, Rathinasamy TK, Inbamani N, Menon T, Kumar SS, Emmadi P, Raghuraman R. Indian J Dent Res. 2011 Jan-Feb;22(1):34-7.

Effect of oil pulling on plaque induced gingivitis: a randomized, controlled, triple-blind study. Asokan S, Emmadi P, Chamundeswari R. Indian J Dent Res. 2009 Jan-Mar;20(1):47-51

Effect of oil pulling on Streptococcus mutans count in plaque and saliva using Dentocult SM Strip mutans test: a randomized, controlled, triple-blind study. Asokan S, Rathan J, Muthu MS, Rathna PV, Emmadi P; Raghuraman; Chamundeswari.
J Indian Soc Pedod Prev Dent. 2008 Mar;26(1):12-7.

Oil pulling therapy. Asokan S. Indian J Dent Res. 2008 Apr-Jun;19(2):169.

Dr. Alex Shvartsman

Due to the immense volume of literature on mercury toxicity and dental mercury, the database of over 11,000 articles and abstracts on mercury toxicity and dental amalgam fillings can be found at http:// dentalwellness4u.com/products/refdoc.htm